PREGNANCY
Health
YOGA

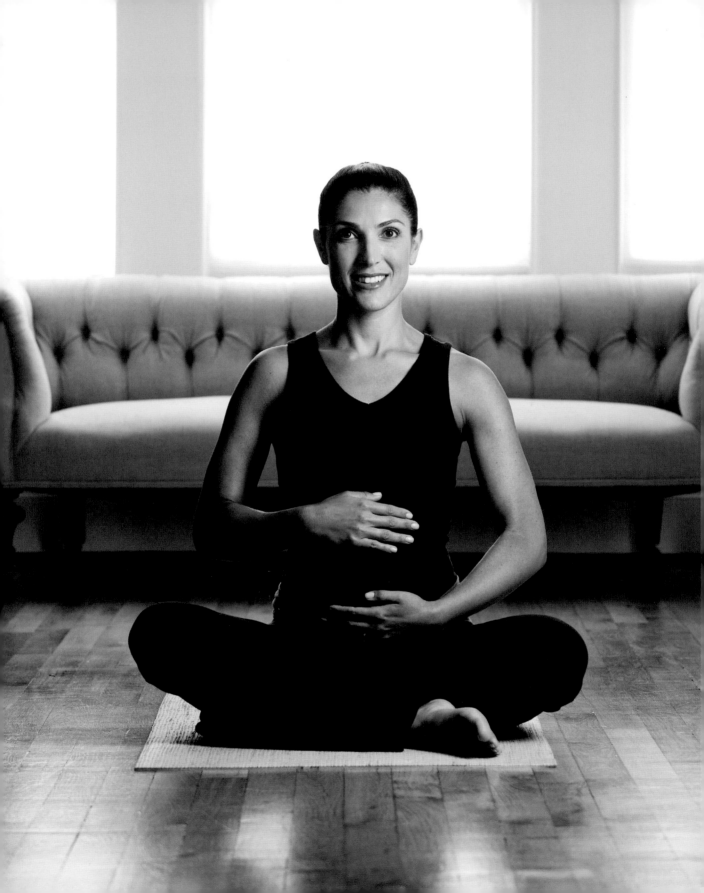

Tara Lee and Mary Attwood

Foreword by Dr Gowri Motha
Creator of the Gentle Birth Method

PREGNANCY
Health
YOGA

Your essential guide for
bump, birth and beyond

DUNCAN BAIRD PUBLISHERS
LONDON

Pregnancy Health Yoga
Tara Lee and Mary Attwood

First published in the United Kingdom and Ireland in 2013 by Duncan Baird Publishers,
an imprint of Watkins Publishing Limited, Sixth Floor, 75 Wells Street, London W1T 3QH

A member of Osprey Group

Managing Editor: Sandra Rigby
Senior Editor: Fiona Robertson
Editor: Jane McIntosh
Managing Designer: Suzanne Tuhrim
Commissioned Photography: Jules Selmes
Make-up Artist: Justine Martin
Pregnancy Yoga Clothing: Designed by Tara Lee for Blossom Mother and Child (www.blossommotherandchild.com)

A CIP record for this book is available from the British Library

ISBN: 978-1-84899-081-4

10 9 8 7 6 5 4 3 2 1

Typeset in Futura, Present and Boundless
Colour reproduction by XY Digital
Printed in China through World Print Ltd

Publisher's note: During your pregnancy, only practise exercises that are suitable for pregnancy. Do not practise
pregnancy yoga before 12–14 weeks of pregnancy and your first scan. It is not advisable to lie flat on your back
after 24 weeks of pregnancy without your upper body being raised higher than your abdomen. It is also not advisable
to practise deep squats after 35 weeks of pregnancy without medical advice. The information in this book is not
intended as a substitute for professional medical advice and treatment. If you are pregnant or are suffering from any
medical conditions or health problems, it is recommended that you consult a medical professional before following
any of the advice or practice suggested in this book. Watkins Publishing Limited, or any other persons who have been
involved in working on this publication, cannot accept responsibility for any injuries or damage incurred as a result
of following the information, exercises or therapeutic techniques contained in this book.

Distributed in the USA and Canada by Sterling Publishing Co., Inc.
387 Park Avenue South, New York, NY 10016-8810

For information about custom editions, special sales, premium and corporate purchases, please contact
Sterling Special Sales Department at 800-805-5489 or specialsales@sterlingpub.com.

CONTENTS

Foreword

Yoga classes during pregnancy have become increasingly popular in the West and this is encouraging because it shows a great willingness on the part of mothers to set aside valuable time to enjoy pregnancy as they prepare for birth. However, teaching yoga to pregnant women can be tremendously challenging because the participants may have a limited range of movements as a result of unsuitable and prolonged sitting positions that we have adopted as the norm in our Western lifestyle.

It takes a very special person with a thorough understanding of human physiology to be able to lead a group of mothers of mixed abilities sensitively in a safe and effective prenatal yoga programme as outlined in this wonderful book. Tara is one such special person who fulfils the necessary criteria in a holistic and artistic manner. Her warm personality engages mothers instantly, ensuring their dedication to the principles and practice of gentle yoga, which encourage a sense of well-being throughout pregnancy and beyond.

Public health research has revealed that reduction of stress in pregnancy not only improves the neurodevelopment of babies in the womb, but also in the immediate neonatal months and in early childhood. Researchers have evaluated and named yoga, massage and listening to music as beneficial activities that reduce stress levels during pregnancy. The practice of yoga during pregnancy has now received recognition as being able to positively enhance the mental and emotional health of our future generations.

My admiration for Tara Lee stems from the fact that she is passionate about supporting pregnant mothers emotionally. This is crucial as pregnancy is a time in a woman's life when mentoring and community support are essential to overall physical and emotional health; they also improve the outcome of pregnancy and birth. Tara's classes bring mothers and babies together into a modern tribal network that supports a balanced approach to pregnancy and birth.

There are numerous physical benefits from yoga during pregnancy: it can help a mother to be stronger physically and energetically; it maximizes her absorption of nutrients by improving overall digestive health; a physically well-nourished and supple mother is able to enjoy pregnancy and recover wonderfully in the postnatal weeks; she will also have the stamina required to offer the constant attention demanded by a newborn baby.

Tara's own confident motherhood gives her an aura of authenticity that inspires pregnant women to embrace motherhood gracefully and look forward to the first tender moments of holding the baby in their arms. Yes! The baby's first touch is the magical moment that ignites the flame of maternal love and instinctual generosity, and enables a new mother to embrace her newborn baby selflessly.

It gives me great pleasure to write the Foreword to this book and to describe the qualities that contribute to Tara's hugely popular pregnancy yoga classes, where mothers rave about her sensitivity, energy and wisdom. The moment you meet this beautiful and remarkable woman you know that you are in the presence of a person who is very clear, very special and divinely inspired. I am delighted to know Tara Lee and even more delighted to know that she is dedicated to sharing her wisdom for years to come with mothers and their families who are fortunate enough to enter her circle of excellence.

Dr Gowri Motha
Creator of the Gentle Birth Method

Introduction

I wrote this book to share the knowledge that I have gained from over a decade of teaching yoga to pregnant women and new mothers and from my own experience as a mother of two. I have seen first hand the positive benefits of yoga practice for pregnancy, for the birthing process and for postnatal recovery, and I am fortunate to have gained so much knowledge from thousands of women about what has worked for them and their babies. I am happy to be able to share this wisdom with you and I hope that you will find this book informative, inspirational and something to treasure.

The step-by-step yoga exercises, visualizations and meditations you will find in this book are all ones that I teach in my classes and are methods that can help in all stages of a woman's transition to motherhood. I am delighted to make these available to everyone through this book.

In our busy society, trying to juggle the demands of a job with those of parenthood can be challenging and time-consuming. The yoga exercises I offer are designed to fit into your daily schedule, to do whenever you can find the time. They are suitable for complete beginners as well as for those who have practised yoga for years.

My style of pregnancy yoga mixes strengthening, dynamic postures with restorative and relaxing ones. I believe that both are important during pregnancy when your energy levels fluctuate from day to day. You can dip into the book and choose the exercises that you feel you need at any given time. Some days – often in the early stages of your pregnancy and just before the birth – you may want to practise a more gentle form of yoga, to give you more energy. On other days, you might feel strong and want to be more active and for these occasions you can select exercises that build strength and stamina. These will improve your fitness levels and help prepare you for labour.

I am often asked how regularly someone should practise yoga and for how long. I usually say practise every day if you can find time, but it is fine if you can only manage a few sessions, or even just one, a week. You will probably find that you feel so revitalized after doing these exercises that you want to do yoga more regularly and for longer. One of the benefits of this book is that you can choose the length of each session. Some days you might get just 10 minutes' practice; on others you might enjoy a full hour and a half. However long you spend, it is a good idea to set aside some time that you know will be just for your yoga.

The ideal practice is a balanced one. Start gently, progressing to stronger postures, and finish with more gentle exercises, including breathing techniques, affirmations, meditation and visualizations. These more creative and insightful routines nourish a vital part of your subconscious and will give you confidence and a more complete experience of this awe-inspiring time.

Tune in to how you feel as you do the exercises in this book. Do them with self-acceptance – without judgment. Enjoy the freedom that you are creating in your mind – the feeling of letting go and of deepening the connection to your baby and yourself.

During yoga we generally breathe through the nose with the mouth closed, unless otherwise stated. Yoga is not about achieving a perfect posture – it is more important to feel than to think through the poses. One of the reasons yoga is so beneficial during pregnancy is that it gets us out of our heads and into our bodies, which helps to bring us into a state that is helpful for labour. When we are able to switch off the thinking part of the brain we allow ourselves to be guided by the wisdom within us. Remember, there is no such thing as the perfect birth – anything can happen, no matter how prepared you are. Accept whatever turn your birth takes, staying open-minded.

The physical exercises in this book are suitable to practise after your 12–14 weeks' scan, assuming you have been given the all-clear from your doctor. Most doctors now recognize that practising yoga and meditation during pregnancy can improve the birthing process, reduce the likelihood of developing backache, hip pain, prolapsed organs, pelvic floor issues and postnatal depression, and improve your general well-being. However, you can use the breathing techniques, visualizations and relaxation poses in this book at any time during your pregnancy.

If you are suffering from a particular condition or have any concerns about your ability to do the exercises in this book, you must check with your doctor that yoga is suitable for you. Always make sure that an exercise is right for you by reading the instructions carefully. In general, listen to your body and if something doesn't feel right or if you feel dizzy, nauseous or experience unusual symptoms or pain, stop the exercise immediately and consult your doctor.

While you do the physical postures wear loose, comfortable clothing. It is preferable to have bare feet. Ideally, start your practice on an empty stomach or after a light snack, such as fruit or some juice. Use a non-slip yoga mat and, if you will be leaning on furniture, make sure it is secure. If sitting cross-legged is uncomfortable for you, try placing a cushion under each knee for support (see below, left) or sit with your legs straight ahead on the floor or kneel. If kneeling is uncomfortable, use a cushion support between your calves and pelvis (see below, right).

I would advise you to read the affirmations, visualizations and meditations in a relaxed state (practising a breathing exercise beforehand can help you get into the right zone), closing your eyes and sitting tall comfortably on a cushion on the floor or on a chair. You can either read the words (out loud or silently) or you can record

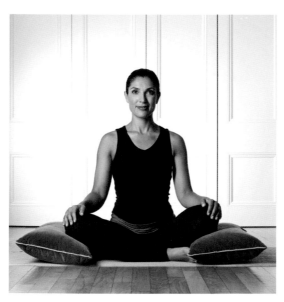

CROSS-LEGGED VARIATION

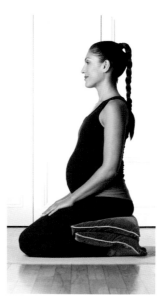

KNEELING VARIATION

them and play them back. Make sure that you are familiar with the breathing techniques and the useful movements for labour so that you feel confident with them and do not need to refer to the book once labour has started.

Pregnancy is just the beginning of the journey into motherhood. Try not to focus only on the birth, as labour is just a stepping stone along the path into your new life. Bear in mind that many of the challenges you will experience during pregnancy are preparing you for the even bigger challenges of motherhood. In *The Prophet*, Kahlil Gibran movingly describes the ideal of a parent as a bow "from which your children as living arrows are sent forth". For the arrow to fly, the bow must be stable. Our children need us, but are independent of us: "You may give them your love but not your thoughts … You may house their bodies but not their souls." It is a reminder that our children are only on loan to us.

Most of all, enjoy this unique time and celebrate the magical journey!

Tara Lee

Know you what it is to be a child?
It is to be something very different from the man of today.
It is to have a spirit yet streaming from the waters of baptism,
It is to believe in love, to believe in loveliness, to believe in belief.
It is to be so little that the elves can reach to whisper in your ear.
It is to turn pumpkins into coaches, and mice into horses,
lowness into loftiness and nothing into everything.
For each child has his fairy godmother in his own soul.
It is to live in a nutshell and count yourself the king of the infinite space;
It is to see a world in a grain of sand,
And a Heaven in a wild flower,
Hold infinity in the palm of your hand,
And eternity in an hour.

Francis Thompson (1859–1907)

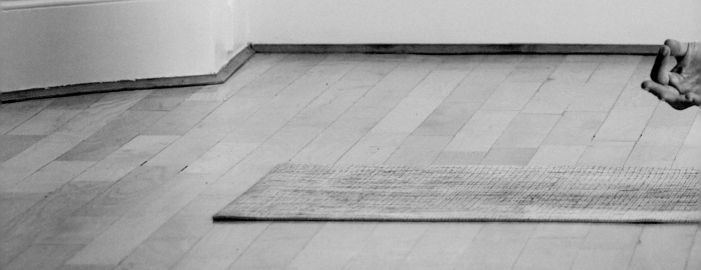
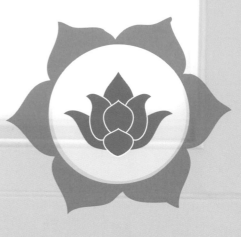

CHAPTER 1
Breathing and Visualization

During pregnancy your emotions can swing from one extreme to another. The breath reflects your mental state, but it can also anchor and support you. Yoga increases awareness and control of breathing, so if you notice that your breath has become shallow because you are stressed, you can use it to bring yourself back into balance. The breath is something you can't leave behind, even if you forget your hospital bag. And if labour starts before you've had time to pack, you will still have your main tool with you – so use it!

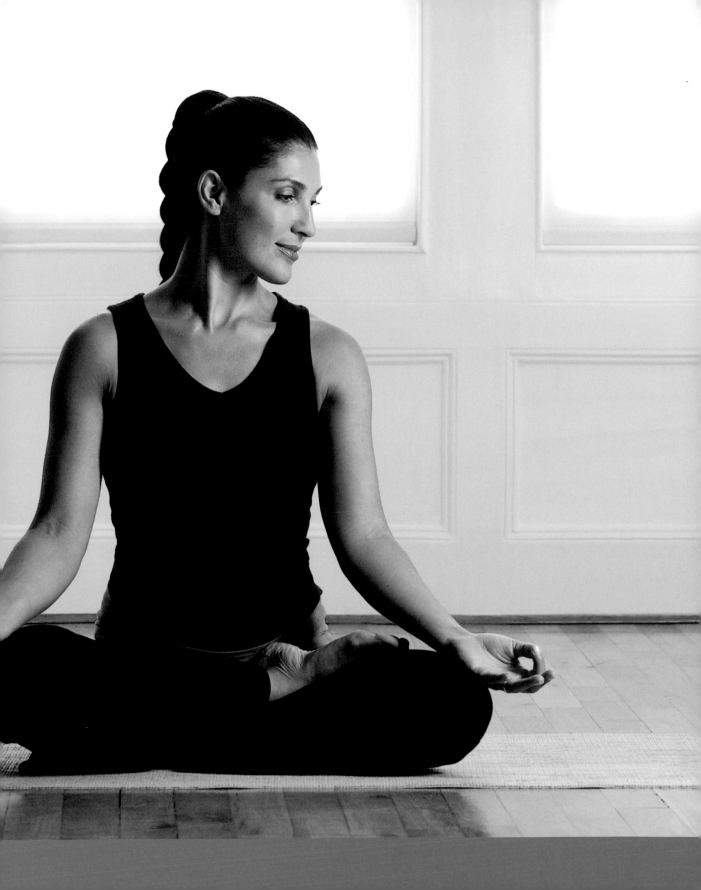

Affirmations

With each breath I send energy to my
baby and the whole of my system.

I breathe deeply to create more space
in my body for my baby.

My breath influences my state of mind.

I alone am responsible for how I breathe.

Breathing deeply, I let go of tension
with each exhalation.

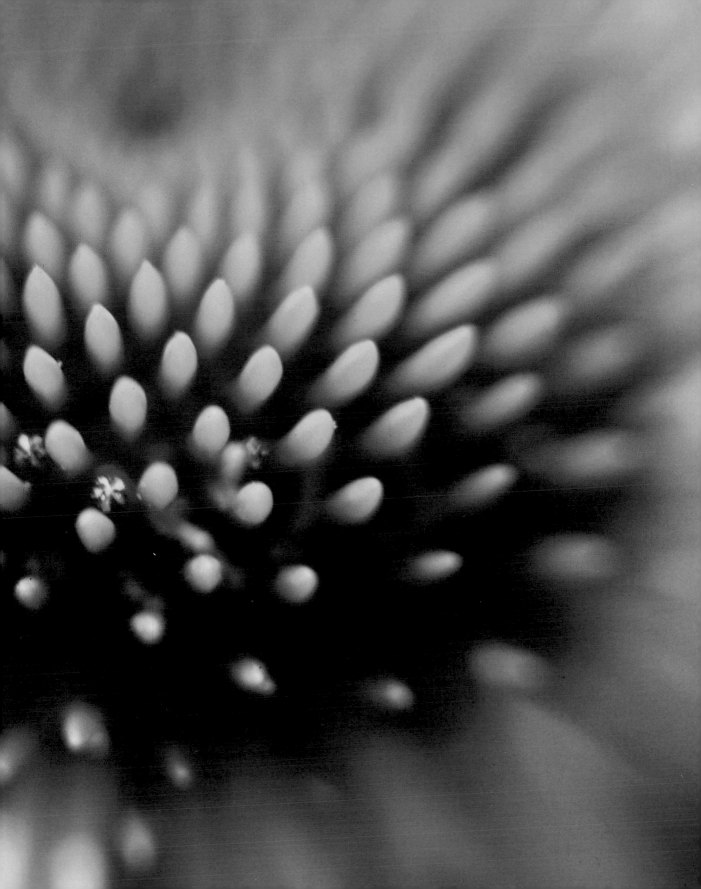

The Power of the Breath

Breath is fundamental to life: the first thing we take when we enter this world and the last thing we take when we leave. Developing an easy, flowing breath is the cornerstone of any yoga practice, but during pregnancy it assumes a special significance. Breathing correctly is a wonderful tool that will empower and energize you – by tuning in to the rhythm of the taking in and the letting go of the breath, you can consciously nurture yourself and your baby.

Gently deepening and slowing the breath and keeping it moving calmly through your body will act as a needle, stitching movement to movement, enriching you and your baby's life-support systems and connecting your physical being with your emotional and spiritual self. Breathing well, and feeling the mind and body responding, can remind us that we are responsible for the way in which we take care of ourselves, but also that we have to let go and trust nature to do the rest.

Learning the simple technique of allowing your breath to flow freely can assist both you and your baby on a number of levels throughout pregnancy as well as during labour and birth. Breathing in a calm, fluid, steady way helps you to move through life in a similar fashion, whereas restricted breath can lead to feelings of being stuck and unable to move forward. The state of your breathing has an impact on and is reflected in every area of life – from your level of confidence and the way you hold yourself to how you relate to others and manage everyday matters.

With yoga we can learn to breathe more deeply, naturally and without effort, and so encourage the vital capacity of the lungs. The quality of our inhalation affects our openness to receive love and joy, to feel fulfilled and to be as comfortable with receiving as with giving. The quality of our exhalation helps us to let go of emotional and physical tensions. We learn to use our breath to tune in to ourselves at a profound level and to find an infinite source of inner support that we can draw on throughout pregnancy and when giving birth.

Inhalation and exhalation can affect your physical, psychological, emotional and spiritual states, as well as your baby's well-being. At its very basic level, breathing sustains the essential biological functions of you and your baby. With an awareness of your breathing you can also directly influence your state of mind and reduce stress throughout pregnancy and while giving birth. The breath can become a tool for you to draw on in any situation to regain a feeling of equilibrium and nurture yourself and your developing child.

In our frantic modern lives we are bombarded with external stimuli saturating the senses. Coming back to the simplicity of the breath helps to calm the mind and allows you to find your own natural rhythm. During pregnancy and birth your senses and emotions are naturally heightened, allowing you to tune in to the inner world of your mind and body more easily. This gift of awareness is also helpful during labour as you become fully attuned to your contractions and your breath in order to facilitate your baby's birth. The shift in focus from the frantic concerns of the world to something that is so simple and basic is a relaxing meditation at your disposal whenever you need it.

Birth Story ...

"We got to the birth centre just in time. I gave birth very soon afterwards in the birthing pool using gas and air, breathing, and the visualization techniques that I had practised in yoga. I won't deny that there were difficult periods during the stronger contractions in the second stage of labour, but by using all of the above to try to keep relaxed and let the body do what it is meant to do, everything became surprisingly manageable. I also remembered to recite one of my favourite birth affirmations: 'With every contraction my baby is coming closer to me.' That really helped to put everything into perspective at the time." *Kate*

Pranayama

Many of us take shallow breaths and rarely expand our lungs to their full capacity; we may even hold our breath when we encounter difficult situations. In this exercise you learn to slow down the breath and breathe deep into the abdomen, helping to reduce the secretion of stress hormones and soothe your baby. Inhaling massages your internal organs as well as your baby; exhaling expels toxins and waste from your system, revitalizing and renewing every cell, and providing energy.

1 Sitting with your legs crossed, rest your hands on your abdomen and close your eyes. Every time you breathe in feel your baby moving up toward your hands and notice whether your breath is shallow in your chest or deep in your abdomen. Deepen and lengthen your breath, and release your shoulders away from your ears. PAUSE Breathing into the abdomen throughout the practice helps to send more oxygen to the baby and makes you feel more centred. Tune in to how you are feeling and notice any stuck or tight areas.

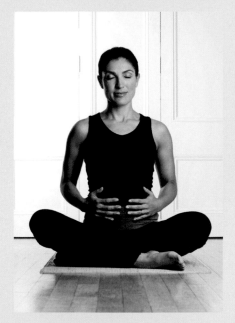

1

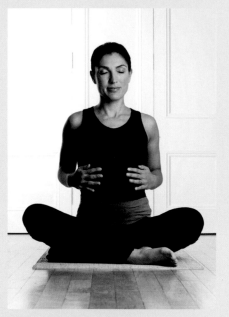

2

Slow down your breathing, direct your breath to those areas of discomfort and notice how your mind and breath can work together to release tension. Sit tall, anchoring down through the hips, lifting up through the spine to create space for your baby. Make sure you aren't holding any tension in your face; keep your eyes soft by relaxing the muscles around your eyes.

2 Place your hands on your ribcage and as you inhale feel your ribcage expand laterally as your fingertips move farther away from each other.

3 As you exhale, feel your fingers move back toward each other. PAUSE 🪷 Inhale, expand; exhale, soften. Listen to the sound of your breath as it moves in and out of your body and feel the movement of the breath creating space in your ribcage.

4 Now bring your fingertips up to rest just beneath your collar bones and breathe into this area, sending the breath into your chest. Make sure your shoulders stay down away from your ears. Send the breath all the way to the top of your lungs as you inhale, and imagine

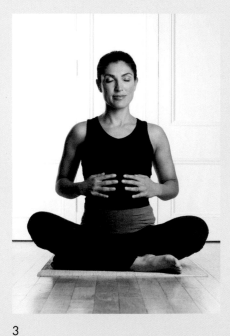

3

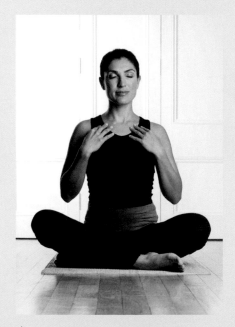

4

emptying them as you exhale. PAUSE 🪷 On the next inhalation imagine the breath moving into the back of your lungs.

5 On your last exhalation bring your hands back down to rest on your baby and see whether your breathing feels a little deeper. PAUSE 🪷 Notice how you feel now. Do you feel more connected to your baby? Do you feel calmer? Is there a sense of stillness within? You may not feel any different, but just notice without judging yourself. Gently massage around your abdomen in a clockwise direction, imagining a golden circle of light around your baby. Now rest one hand on the heart centre and the other on your navel below the belly button and feel the breath moving in your body. PAUSE 🪷 With each breath imagine sending positive energy to your baby. Feel a connection from your heart to your baby's heart, sending love to your baby.

6 Now slowly open your eyes again, keeping your gaze soft and your face relaxed.

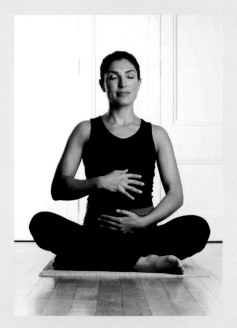

5

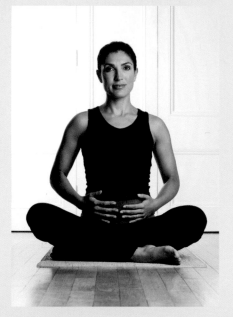

6

Alternate Nostril Breathing

Alternate Nostril Breathing helps to balance masculine and feminine energy (see page 22) and calms, relaxes and refreshes all aspects of your mind and body. It can also help with insomnia. Avoid if you have severe nasal congestion.

1 Sit cross-legged. With eyes closed, take a deep breath in.

2 Close your right nostril with your right thumb, keeping your left nostril open. Inhale through the left nostril, then close it with the ring finger, release the thumb and exhale through the right nostril.

3 Inhale through the right nostril, then close it with the thumb, release the ring finger and exhale through the left nostril. Repeat Steps 2 and 3 for 1–2 minutes.

4 Keep the breath slow and relaxed, with in-breaths and out-breaths of similar length. Finish by exhaling through the left nostril to activate the feminine, lunar, calming and cooling energy.

5 Release your hand to your right knee and keep your eyes closed. Feel the breath moving more evenly through both nostrils now as you breathe deeply for a minute or longer. Slowly open your eyes when you feel ready.

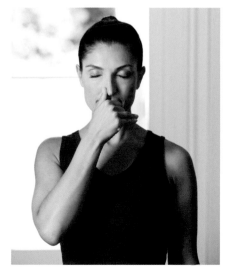

2

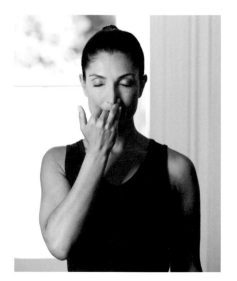

3

Bellow Breathing

The Alternate Nostril Breathing exercise on page 21 acts on the subtle body by opening up and purifying the channels of energy known in Sanskrit as *nadis*. It strengthens the nervous system and aligns the two sides of the brain by regulating masculine energy, associated with the right nostril, and feminine energy, associated with the left nostril. The exercise acts as a great emotional leveller, helping to correct the imbalances that can occur during pregnancy.

In contrast, Bellow Breathing provides relief from one of the physical changes associated with pregnancy. As the womb expands, especially in the later stages, the internal organs become compressed and many women feel rib pain and shortness of breath. One of the biggest benefits of practising yoga and yogic breathing (particularly Bellow Breathing) during pregnancy is that it helps to create more space in the abdomen to accommodate your growing baby.

1 Sitting tall, start by interlacing your fingers under your chin, keeping your elbows down.

2 Inhale through the nose, lifting your elbows high with palms down, and imagine filling your lungs with breath-like bellows.

3 Exhale through the nose, lowering your elbows back down toward each other and emptying out your lungs.

4 Again inhale, elbows rising, breathing all the way up to your armpits, then release your elbows back down as you exhale slowly.

5 Now, as you inhale, see if you can find an extra 10 percent of room at the top of the breath and then exhale, letting go, emptying all the breath. PAUSE 🪷 On the in-breath notice the space you are creating in your body as your lungs fully expand, and the deep cleansing that comes with the exhalation. Repeat 3 more times.

6 This time as you inhale breathe in through your nose and as you exhale breathe out steadily through your mouth, blowing the breath away. Repeat gently 3 more times.

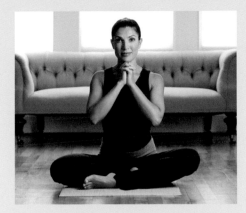

3

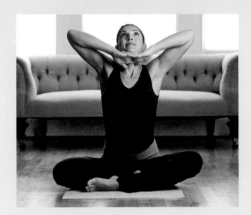

2

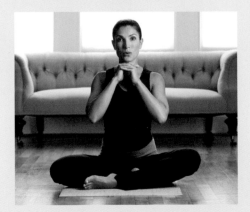

1

Adding Sound to Breathing

In this practice you will synchronize movement with the breath, adding sounds. When you add sound to the exhalation, it helps to lengthen the out-breath and gives the muscles more time to release, which will be helpful for labour and release mood-boosting endorphins. Sound also helps you to lose your inhibitions – this can improve your experience of labour. Your baby can hear and feel your voice from as early as 16 weeks in the womb. Visualizing sounds moving down your body to your baby bathes your baby in a pool of vibration and will help your energy to move downward, assisting the birth.

1 You can perform this exercise standing or seated. Start with your hands resting on your belly and notice how you are feeling. Breathing in deeply with palms turned upward by your sides, bring your palms to prayer pose in front of your heart and allow your arms to float up.

2 Let your palms meet above your head at the top of your inhalation.

3 Slowly exhaling, float your arms back down (palms down) so your hands reach the floor by the end of the breath.

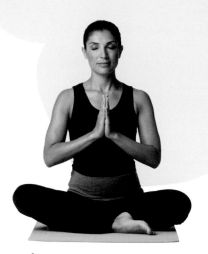

1

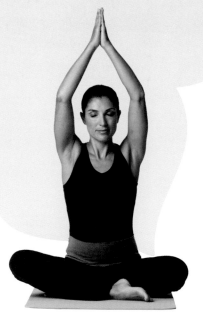

2

4 Inhale and let your arms float back up. Feel the space between your shoulders and your ears and allow your breath to guide the movement. Keep your breath fluid and don't hold it at any time (your breath is an indicator of your state of mind). Release your arms back down.

5 Inhale, still breathing only through the nose, and lift your arms back up again. Now you will add sound to the movement – making a low "AAH" sound when releasing your arms back down. Notice how much longer the exhalation lasts when using sounds. Repeat this 3 times.

6 Now bring your arms down through the centre line, palms touching, making the sound "OM" (in three parts: "aaa" "oooo" "mmmm"). Your baby can hear and feel this vibration.

7 Place your hands back on your belly, close your eyes and reflect on how you feel now. Notice a sense of inner vibration that still remains.

8 Bring one hand up to your heart and place the other on your navel below your belly button. PAUSE 🪷 Feel the bond of love between you and your baby and give gratitude to life for this miracle growing within you.

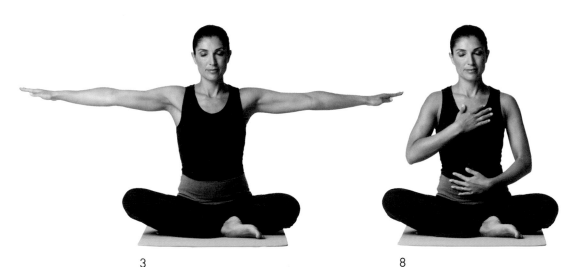

3

8

CHAPTER 2
Creating Space

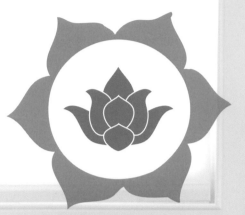

Being pregnant means that you need to create space in a number of different areas – on a purely physical level your body has to expand to accommodate a growing baby, but you also need to make mental and emotional adjustments in preparation for an important new person entering your life. Your posture and how you move can directly affect the health of your internal organs and the way you feel, so keeping a sense of space in your torso benefits both you and your baby. Yoga is one of the best forms of practice for creating space in every aspect of your life because it is all-encompassing, working on a number of levels.

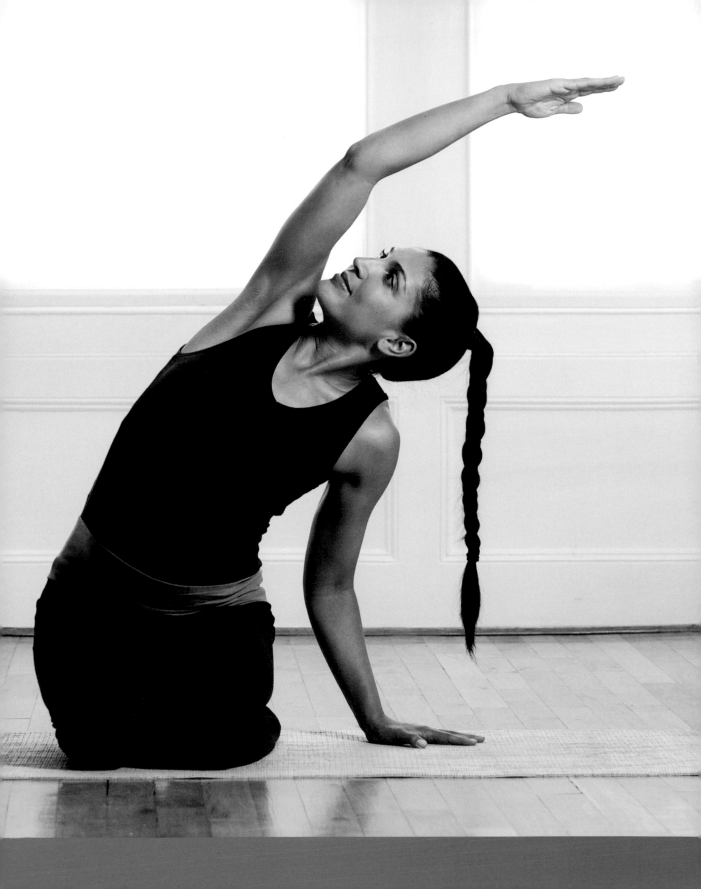

Affirmations

I breathe deeply and sit tall so that I can create more space for me and my baby.

I focus on my breathing to create more space and calm in my mind.

By sitting taller I feel more energized and more positive.

I transfer lightness, peace and joy to my baby.

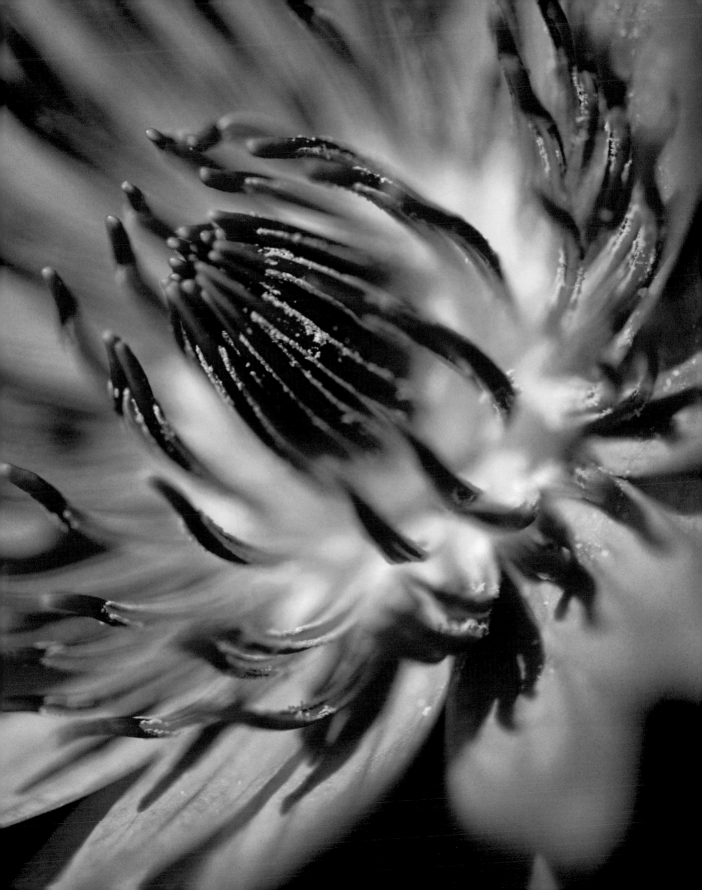

The Need for Space

When women discover they are pregnant they may experience a variety of emotions, such as excitement, surprise, shock or fear. Many struggle to get to grips with the idea of carrying a new life and all the changes that this might entail emotionally and physically. In order to embrace the enormous changes taking place inside, we need to make space in our bodies and our minds.

If you are in the last few weeks of pregnancy and it feels like there's no room left in your upper abdomen, don't worry – as your baby starts to descend into your pelvis, the area around the ribcage will be freed up and you should feel much more comfortable. It is common to feel rib pain particularly toward the end of the second trimester and throughout the third trimester until the baby drops. Rib pain occurs because the internal organs become compressed by the top of the uterus as your baby grows. To alleviate discomfort, there are exercises in this chapter that extend and strengthen your side and waist muscles, creating more space in your torso.

In Chinese medicine the expansion of the womb as a baby grows during pregnancy is connected to the opening of the heart, which perhaps offers some insight as to why women can become more emotional in pregnancy. In yoga philosophy, the expressions of the body have their equivalent in the mind. During pregnancy the hormone relaxin loosens joints, muscles and ligaments; this softening is mirrored in our hearts and we also become more centred. We recognize our own vulnerability and, like a lioness defending her young, we want to protect ourselves and our growing baby. Everything we do needs to be conducted with awareness and respect for our centre, which has shifted both physically and emotionally.

We all need to create more space from time to time. This might involve removing clutter from our immediate environment, or retreating to a less busy place for a holiday, or just staring into the distance and letting our mind escape from a torrent of busy thoughts. When we meditate, we allow the mind to release its daily preoccupations and be calm. Meditation enables us to slip into a space where time and location are suspended and this holds numerous health benefits for both the physical and the subtle bodies. It gives us room to rejuvenate – as we are not touched by the harsh demands of time, body functions slow down and the ageing process is suspended temporarily. Your baby will enjoy a blissful state of calm through your experience.

Creating space in our minds through yoga helps us to appreciate the amazing fact that a separate being is growing within us. We have little control over this process but we can choose what we eat and drink in order to nourish our baby physically as best we can. It is also important to nurture the baby with positive emotions and this we can do through creating space in our lives for mindfulness, meditation, visualization and yoga. Our body is a vessel for our baby yet we can still retreat to a sanctuary within ourselves. We can use this time to connect with our inner self and to develop the bond with our unborn baby. Yoga can create space where there was compression, can make open what was closed and can make soft our hard and abrasive edges. The process of pregnancy itself opens and expands our hearts and our capacity to love.

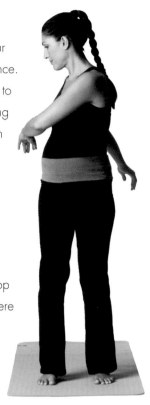

Birth Story ...

"Tara's classes made me feel so good throughout pregnancy and really helped to prepare me for my son's birth. Whenever I was feeling uncomfortable, yoga gave me a feeling of more space in my body and made me feel calmer. It also aided me in accepting the changes I was experiencing and provided space for my thoughts. I found that the meditation techniques in combination with my yoga practice definitely helped to make the whole labour and birth very calm. I had been quite nervous about how I would cope, but when it came to it I drew on those lessons of movement and breathing and felt positive and confident throughout." Andrea

Meditation for Creating Space in the Mind

We frequently get so caught up in bringing organization to our lives that we find it hard just to "be". Creating space between our thoughts allows us to experience a different reality. Meditation is one way to achieve this.

1 Sit comfortably on a cushion with your legs crossed or kneel if you have any groin pain. Either place both hands on your baby or support your lower back by pressing one hand gently there if you have backache.

2 Close your eyes, soften the muscles of your face and keep your jaw relaxed, breathing steadily in and out through your nostrils. Slow down and deepen your breath. See if you can grow taller through the spine and feel the support of the floor beneath you. Grow from that support, lengthening upward through the spine. PAUSE ✿ Imagine that you are creating space between each of your vertebrae with each breath. Imagine that your spine is like a necklace of prayer beads with a space between each bead. Imagine that you are creating more room for your baby and space for you to feel more comfortable.

3 Feel strength and support from the back of your body so that you can start to lift upward out of the front of your body. Feel the space between each rib, as you breathe laterally, and feel that space gradually increasing with each breath.

4 As you slow down and focus on the rhythmic sound of your breath, become aware of the natural pause at the end of each exhalation, before your next breath starts. Notice the pause at the top of your inhalation, before the exhalation starts. PAUSE ✿ Do you feel a sense of freedom now as you breathe more openly, without so much resistance? With this freedom in the breath, can you feel a sense of growing space in your mind as your thoughts start to slow down and you begin to feel more present, living in this moment? It is almost as if time is suspended as you continue to slow

your breath, effortlessly, focusing on the sound and sensation of the breath, feeling a connection to the present. Nothing else matters except this moment ... now you feel calm, present, connected to your body and connected to your baby. You feel peaceful and content with where you are in this moment and you feel an immense gratitude to your body for producing and growing this miracle of life within you. You trust that your body knows exactly what to do and that you have an innate wisdom that will take you through pregnancy and the birth of your baby.

5 Stay here for a few more minutes, still focusing on the feeling of space you have created in your mind and body. Keeping your eyes closed, start to slowly bring your awareness back into the room you are in. PAUSE Imagine connecting to your baby beneath your hand and smile as though your baby could also feel this smile and experience a warm feeling inside.

6 When you feel ready, slowly open your eyes and stretch your legs in front of you, giving them a good shake. Sit tall, keeping a sense of spaciousness throughout your body.

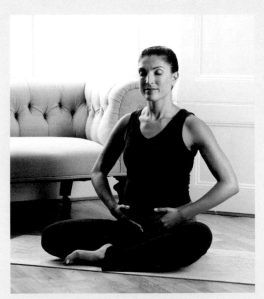

1

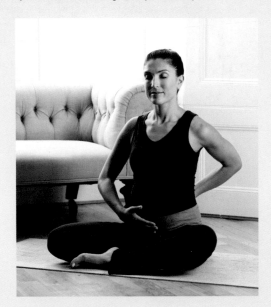

1 VARIATION

Correct Seated Posture

When practising any seated exercises it's always good to remember your posture. Make sure that you are not overarching your back or slouching. It's easy to forget this, especially as your baby grows and becomes heavier. If you can maintain a correct posture when sitting this will help your baby to remain in a good position ready for birth and keep your internal organs functioning healthily. Maintaining correct posture when you are sitting is also good for your spine.

CORRECT

Sit comfortably and feel your buttock bones connecting with the floor. Gently rock your pelvis back and forth until you find a neutral place to rest. Imagine that you are sending your tailbone down to the floor, keeping a sense of lengthening down through the spine. Your back should be long and not leaning forward or backward (see right, top). Continue to practise correct sitting whenever possible.

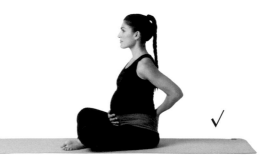

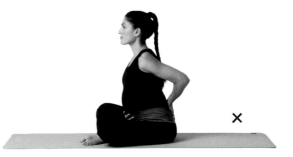

INCORRECT

Make sure you are not tilting forward (see right, centre). This can create lordosis (an inward curve) in the spine. Also avoid rounding your upper back with your body leaning back (see right, bottom).

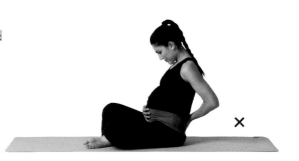

Lengthening the Torso

Shortness of breath is common in pregnancy and hunching or slouching only make the problem worse. The stretch in this exercise allows your lungs to expand so you can breathe fully and deeply.

1 Sit cross-legged (supporting your knees with cushions, if necessary). If you find this uncomfortable, kneel with your buttocks on your heels. With palms facing down, interlace your fingers.

2 As you inhale lift your arms above your head, keeping your shoulders relaxed.

3 On the next in-breath release your head back, look up to your hands, then exhale and lower the chin to the chest, feeling the stretch through your neck.

4 Inhale, looking up, and reach your arms a bit farther back if you can. Exhale with your chin tucked under, keeping the back of your neck long. Repeat 3 more times.

5 Inhale once more, filling your lungs, and as you exhale release your arms down and rest. PAUSE Allow your breath to fill your lungs and visualize the extra space you have created throughout your torso for yourself and your growing baby.

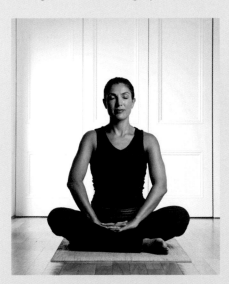

1

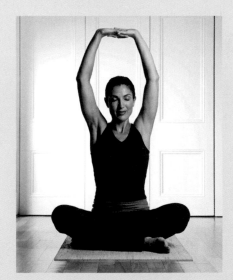

2

Kneeling Side Stretches

Use this exercise to create space between the small muscles in the ribcage, which often get compressed during pregnancy.

1 Kneeling or sitting cross-legged, place your right hand on the floor by your side and, as you inhale, lift your left arm diagonally over your ear. Keep grounded down through the right hip and look straight ahead. Exhale and come back to the centre.

2 Place your right hand down again and repeat the stretch 3–5 times, inhaling as your arm comes up, exhaling as you bring it down. With each repetition start to lengthen the stretch, keeping your left shoulder and your chest open toward the ceiling. Imagine breathing into your left lung and remember to keep elongating the stretch. Keep both sit bones rooted to the floor, if possible.

3 Place your left hand on the floor and repeat Steps 1 and 2, stretching the right side of your body. As before, try to reach a little farther each time with the top arm and keep your shoulder down, away from your ear.

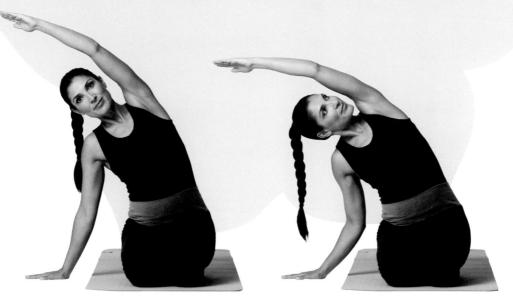

1

2

Baddha Konasana

Baddha Konasana strengthens the muscles of the pelvic region and lower back, and soothes back pain. It can also help the pelvis to broaden, providing more space and preparing you for birth. This powerful pose should be avoided if you are suffering from any groin pain or symphisis pubic dysfunction (SPD).

Sit with the soles of your feet touching (but not too close to your pelvis, to avoid over-stretching the ligaments). Feel the stretch in your inner thighs. (Placing cushions as support under your knees will ease the stretch.)

• You can also practise this pose lying down. If you are over 25 weeks pregnant, make sure your chest is higher than your abdomen. With your back supported, the pelvic region and thoracic diaphragm are able to release. Lying here can also help you to lengthen your exhalation, relaxing your mind. Remember to roll over to one side when you get up from a lying-down position to avoid any strain. Place your opposite hand on the floor or bed, press into it and roll gently up (see below, bottom right).

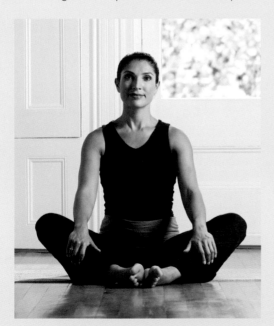

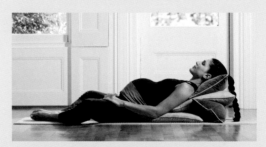

VARIATION

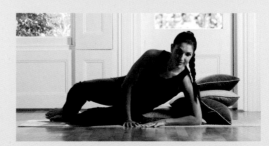

HOW TO GET UP SAFELY

Arm Stretches on All Fours

Being in an all-fours position gives your baby plenty of space and takes the pressure off your back and pelvis. Optimal foetal positioning is a key factor in making labour and birth easier, so if your baby is in a transverse, breech or posterior position, encourage it to turn by spending as much time as possible on your hands and knees. This exercise is a great way of moving the weight of your baby out of your pelvis and into the front of your body, creating space in your torso and releasing your lower back. If you feel dizzy or need to rest during this or any other exercise, remember to move into Child's Pose (see pages 80–81) and breathe deeply.

1 Move onto all fours. Position your knees wider than your hips to make a more stable base (unless you have groin pain). PAUSE 🪷

- If you have wrist pain or carpal tunnel syndrome, rest on your forearms (see opposite, bottom left) or put a cushion under your wrists, to relieve pressure.

- If you have any pain in your wrists, you can also elevate your hands using blocks or books to relieve some of the pressure. Fan out your fingers, making sure the middle fingers point forward, and press down through the knuckles. You can rest here and breathe, or you can try the variation for Step 2.

- If you have any pain in your knees you can roll your mat for extra cushioning or put a pillow underneath your knees for extra support.

2 Move your right hand a little toward your left hand and extend your left arm up as far as possible, opening the left side of your body and ribcage. If you can, follow your arm with your gaze (if you have neck problems, keep looking down). PAUSE 🪷

- If you have wrist pain, place one book on top of another at the centre of the mat and raise your arm (see opposite, bottom right). This extra elevation will help you to rotate, opening your ribcage without straining your back.

3 Exhale as you lower your arm. Inhaling, repeat with your right arm. Exhale, release and repeat three times on each side. Keep pressing down through your supporting hand into the mat, spreading out your fingers.

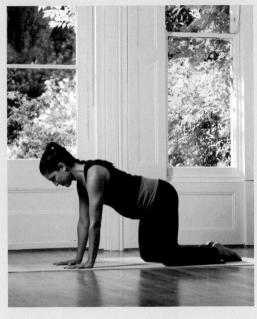

1

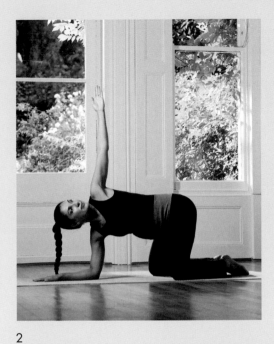

2

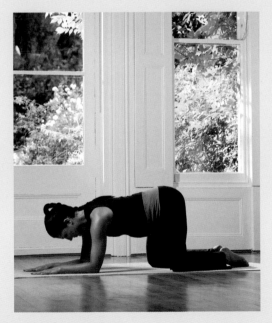

1 VARIATION

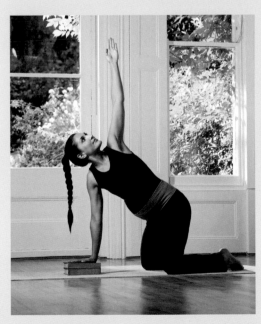

2 VARIATION

Kneeling and Standing Stretch

Helpful if you are feeling stiff after sitting for a long time, this stretch lengthens the spine and takes the weight of your baby forward, giving it more room.

1 Kneel about 2ft (50cm) away from the wall with knees wide enough apart so you feel stable. Walk your hands as high up the wall as you can and sink your chest toward the wall.

2 Breathe in, then exhale, sinking your chest toward the wall, opening the middle of your back. PAUSE 🪷 Enjoy the sense of lightness. If you feel any discomfort in your lower back gently come out of the stretch. Otherwise stay here for 5–10 breaths. Gently walk your hands down the wall and release the stretch.

3 Stand at a distance away from the wall and place your hands on it to make a right angle with your body and legs. Press back through your heels and move your hips back away from the wall while pressing into it with your hands. Feel a stretch in the backs of your legs and your waist. Hold for 5–10 breaths. Bend your knees and walk toward the wall to release.

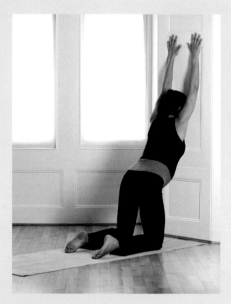

1

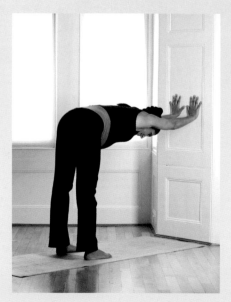

3

Arm Swinging

This is a relaxed movement where you should experience a sense of freedom and space in the body. You can use it to imagine getting rid of unwanted tension, emotions or anxieties, and it also helps to cool you down.

1 With your hips forward and knees bent, swing your arms from side to side. Twist from the upper back, keeping your hips square. Close your eyes (unless you feel dizzy) and enjoy this release. Breathe in a relaxed way and allow the freeness of this movement to transfer to your mind, encouraging it to let go of unwanted thoughts.

2 Feel the space in your upper body as you gently sway, feeling free. Slow down the swinging gradually as you come back to the centre.

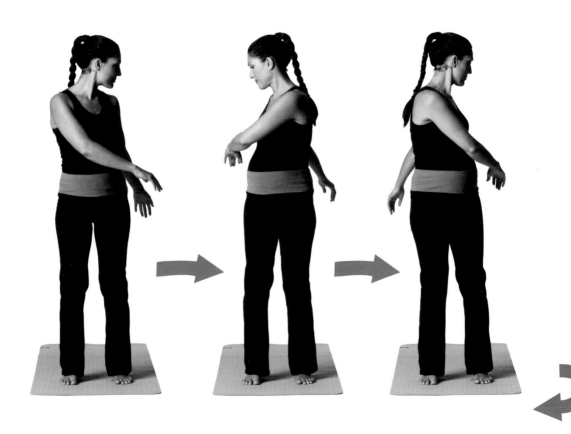

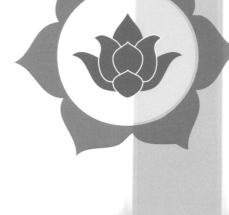

CHAPTER 3
Strength and Stamina

Pregnancy takes us on an amazing journey and, like all new experiences, this can sometimes be a little daunting – but yoga can help us to cope when we are out of our comfort zone. If we treat ourselves with care and respect, we can push our boundaries and build our strength and stamina. This will increase our self-confidence and help the body become more able to let go, in turn enabling the mind to release tension and negativity.

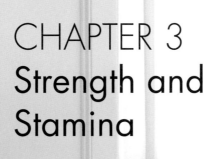

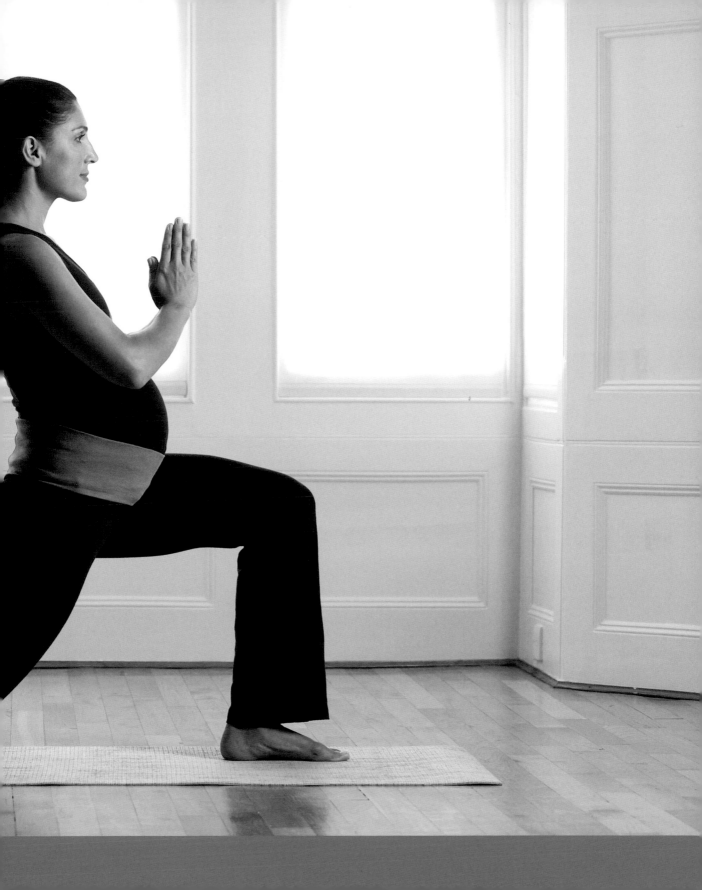

Affirmations

My body is strong, my mind is strong.

I remain positive and strong throughout
my pregnancy and labour.

I gather strength from the support
around and within me.

Whatever direction my labour takes, my
breathing will help me to stay strong and focused.

I will recover quickly because I am fit and strong.

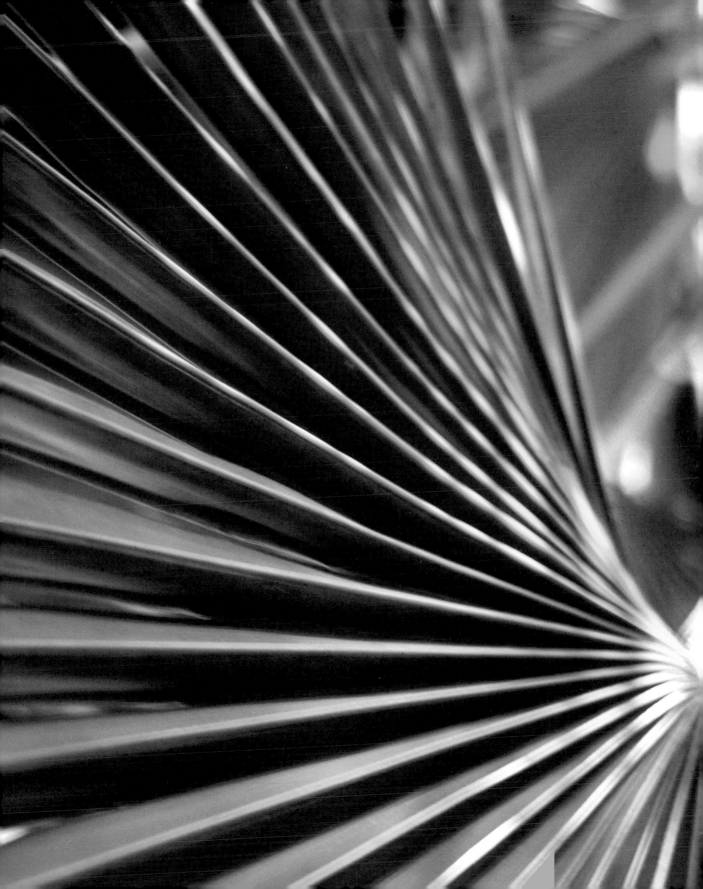

Feeling Strong and Energetic

Developing and maintaining strength and stamina throughout pregnancy has many important benefits. The idea that pregnancy is a time when you become increasingly weak and tired does not have to be true. Many women discover a new relationship with themselves and feel strong throughout their pregnancy. Being pregnant focuses attention on ourselves and makes us consider lifestyle choices, such as our working, eating and exercise habits. If you are not feeling energetic or healthy, you may need to think about making some changes in these areas, in addition to your pregnancy yoga routine.

Energy is something that you need throughout your pregnancy. Feeling tired affects us deeply – the body becomes lethargic and our thoughts and aspirations may also become apathetic. Developing reserves of strength will help you during labour and birth and stand you in good stead when it comes to satisfying the demands of a new baby. Unlike other forms of exercise, yoga will not deplete your energy levels. There are no forceful or pounding movements to put pressure on your joints and tire your muscles. Your cells will be renewed at the deepest level so you feel revitalized after practice. During pregnancy, your body movements can become more restricted, so practising yoga can also bring a sense of flexibility and lightness.

As your baby becomes heavier, you will need to strengthen your muscles to support the extra weight. A strong lower back and core will help prevent back pain caused by the forward and downward pull of your baby. A strong body also increases self-confidence. Your attitude will be more positive and you will feel better equipped to handle whatever comes your way. You wouldn't enter a marathon without any training so make time for exercise and yoga practice – that way, if you happen to have a long labour, you will be as mentally and physically prepared as possible. Also, if you are fit, your recovery from birth – whether natural or a C-section – is likely to be a lot quicker.

If you find yourself lacking in energy during pregnancy, this may be a sign that you need a rest or a change of diet. You should also ask your doctor to check that your iron levels are high enough. Light exercise, such as yoga, a walk or a swim, can revitalize you. If you feel tired while practising yoga, this may simply be due to its cleansing effects, flushing toxins from your body. Persist and you will find that your energy levels are very soon renewed.

Remember that life consists of ebb and flow and that it is important to maintain energetic balance – for example, activity and rest, action and contemplation, strength and softness. Energy can lie dormant, but if you tune in to your body you may find that you experience an increased flow of energy and creativity during your pregnancy.

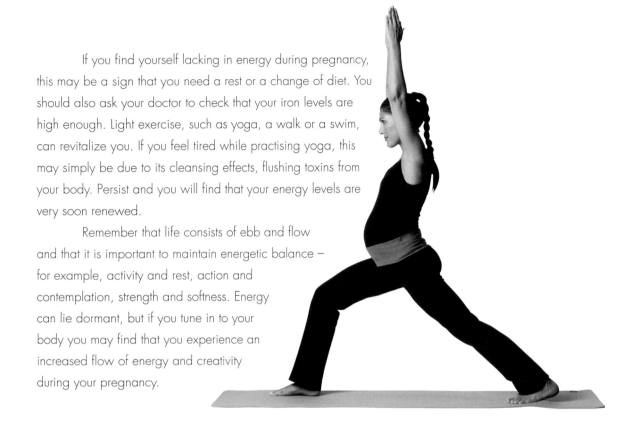

Birth Story ...

"I arrived at the birthing centre feeling very tense, but then all the lessons I had learned from Tara in my yoga classes started to flood into my mind. I knelt down on all fours and started rocking my body back and forth ... It had been five and half hours since labour started and I was getting tired and, although my baby's head was showing, when I stopped pushing he would go back inside. This went on for 30 minutes, so the midwife moved me onto a birthing stool. I pushed again, and this time at the end of the push I let out an enormous out-breath. I performed this amazing and powerful action three times and our beautiful baby boy was born." Viva

Cat and Swooping Cat

This is a wonderful exercise for strengthening and toning the arms. It also increases flexibility and blood flow around the spine and in general is one of the most beneficial exercises you can do for your back. If you have backache, try practising Cat and Swooping Cat for just a few minutes every day and you'll soon notice the difference.

1 Start on all fours in a neutral position. With your hands and knees on the floor, make sure that your shoulders are directly above your wrists. You can move your knees slightly farther apart than your hips.

2 Inhale, and then as you breathe out, tuck the pelvis under as if hugging your baby toward you. Allow your head to drop, bring your chin toward your chest and round up through your shoulders and upper back. Press down through all your fingers, keeping the knuckles down.

3 Inhaling, bring your spine to a neutral position, extending through the crown of your head. Keep your gaze directed down between your hands. You want to lengthen from the crown of the head to the tailbone without letting your lower back collapse.

4 Repeat Steps 1–3 (3–5 times) and then, if you find this sequence easy, you can enhance the movement with the Swooping Cat as follows.

5 Open your knees a bit wider, inhale through the nose, then exhale bending the elbows as you bring the hips back, keeping your chin tucked in and your spine rounded. As you sink farther back your arms will straighten.

6 Inhale, swooping the body forward with the chest low.

7 Press your hands into the floor as you lift back up.

8 Continue swooping back and forth fluidly in a wave-like movement, moving with the breath. Gradually build up your strength, repeating Steps 5–8, aiming for 5 rounds. Rest whenever you need to.

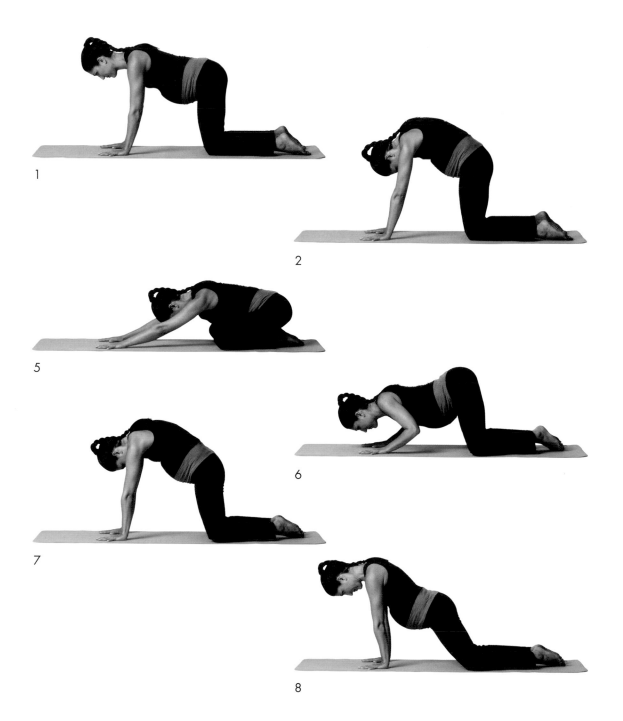

1

2

5

6

7

8

Lion Breath

Practising Lion Breath after Cat and Swooping Cat can feel empowering as it symbolizes courage and strength as well as helping to cleanse the lungs. It relieves facial tension and allows the jaw to release. Being on all fours helps to position your baby for the birth and gives you stability during contractions.

As you strongly exhale through your mouth, stick out your tongue, expel all the air from your lungs and allow your eyes to gaze upward. Then, with mouth closed, inhale through your nose and relax your gaze. You can repeat this 3–5 times.

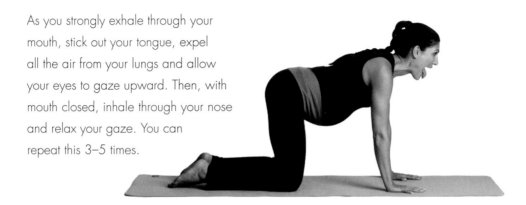

Strengthening the Pelvic Floor

To locate your pelvic floor, imagine the muscle you would use to stop the flow of urine. During pregnancy, your pelvic floor can become weakened by the hormone relaxin and the weight of the baby. It is essential to strengthen this area, as weakness here can lead to stress incontinence. A strong pelvic floor can help to shorten the second stage of labour, and you will also need to know how to release these muscles for the birth. Try to do this exercise every day during pregnancy and especially after the birth, even if you have had a caesarean.

1 Kneel on all fours and move your hands slightly forward from your shoulders, resting your forehead on your hands with your hips high. (If this position is uncomfortable you can sit cross-legged.) Inhale and squeeze and lift your pelvic floor, then release on the exhale. Repeat this a few more times.

2 Keep your jaw relaxed. This time reverse the breathing. Try to squeeze as you exhale and release as you inhale. Repeat 10 times.

3 Now squeeze, lift and hold for 5 counts. Breathe normally, then release. One more time, squeeze, lift and hold for 5 slow counts, then release. Repeat 3 more times and notice whether you are able to keep lifting your pelvic floor muscle for 5 slow counts. Practise until you are able to do this.

4 Now imagine that you are going in a lift up to the first floor as you squeeze a little. Move up to the second floor as you squeeze a little higher. Go all the way to the top floor still holding and

squeezing as high as you can. Release a little, down to the second floor; release a little more to the first floor; and then release completely back down to the ground floor. Repeat at your own pace and make sure you are connecting to your deep, internal muscles. Keep the jaw as relaxed as possible. On the last round imagine you are coming all the way down to the basement, completely letting go. If you are unable to control the lowering in stages – if it all comes crashing down in one go! – it's particularly important to practise regularly.

5 Now relax your pelvic floor and either come back up or rest in Child's Pose (see pages 80–81).

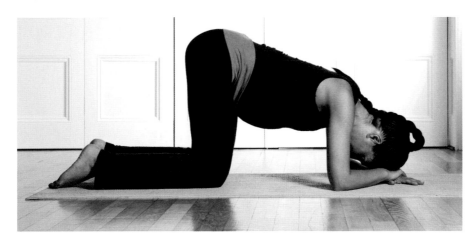

Sitting on Heels with Toes Tucked Under

This is an intense stretch for the toes and bottoms of the feet. As pregnancy progresses it becomes more and more important to look after all aspects of your being. The feet are often neglected – and yet they have to carry us and our growing babies for every step of our journey. This exercise develops a feeling of groundedness on both a physical and an emotional plane. It stretches out the balls of the feet and the toes, which in reflexology and Traditional Chinese Medicine correspond to the lungs, so enjoy the opening of the whole of your body. Notice how focusing on your breathing lessens discomfort – a useful tool for labour.

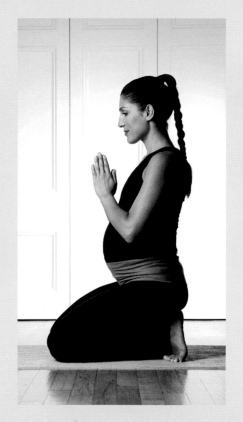

1 Sit back on your heels, tucking your toes underneath you. Bring your palms together in front of your chest in prayer pose. Your knees shouldn't hurt but there may be an intense feeling in your toes. Have faith – they won't break!

2 Try to keep your spine straight – don't collapse your middle back. Breathe deeply through the discomfort in your feet and focus your mind to send your breath into that area.

3 Keep breathing, directing the breath into the area of discomfort and stay there for 5–10 breaths.

Chair

This pose is great for building strength in the legs to carry the weight of your baby. It is also a very grounding posture, rooting you to the earth. It strengthens the lower body while opening the shoulders and chest, and can be helpful for flat feet. You can use a wall for support if you prefer.

1 Stand in *Tadasana* (see page 55) with your feet hip-width apart or wider for stability. Feel the grounding through your feet, sending energy down through your legs.

2 As you inhale reach your arms up above your head, keeping your shoulders down. Exhale and bend your knees, keeping your thighs parallel. Sink low (don't let your hips go lower than your knees) and imagine you are sitting in a chair, but slightly tuck the tailbone under to keep the lower back long. Aim for 5 slow breaths, feeling the strength building in your legs.

3 To come out of this position, inhale and straighten your legs, then exhale, releasing the arms down to your sides.

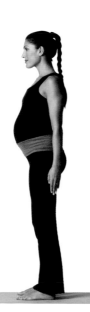

1

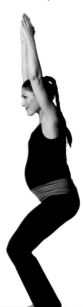

2

Correct and Incorrect Standing Positions

It is especially important to pay attention to good posture during pregnancy, when the weight of your baby may cause your pelvis to tilt, overarching your lower back and leading to back pain.

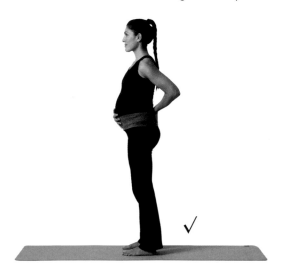

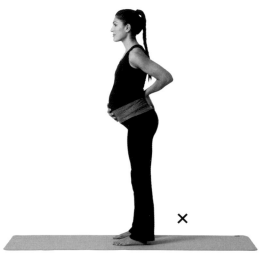

CORRECT
Stand with your feet parallel, hip-width apart or a little wider, and weight even through both feet. The back of your neck should be long, your chin level to the ground. Do not tilt your pelvis. Tuck your tailbone slightly under or send it down toward the floor to lengthen your lower back. Your shoulder blades should gently move down and back. Draw up through your pelvic floor and draw your tummy muscles in slightly to stand taller.

INCORRECT
Because you are carrying more weight at the front of your body – from your growing breasts and belly – your centre of gravity is farther forward, making your lower back overarch as your pelvis tips forward. Your upper back and shoulders round and your hips and chest tighten.

Tadasana

Tadasana means "mountain" in Sanskrit, symbolizing strength and expressing the duality of being rooted to the earth while reaching to great heights. If you practise this posture whenever you can, your body will remember it and it will become "second nature" to you.

Standing tall, feet hip-width apart and toes facing forward, extend up through your spine to the crown of your head. Reach your arms down by your sides and send energy through your fingers. Lift up through your thighs, engaging the muscles without locking your knees, feeling strong through your legs. Lengthen your tailbone and try not to collapse into your lower back. Bring your awareness through your feet, spread out your toes and feel strongly connected to the earth. Lift up through your spine and through the whole front of your body. PAUSE 🪷 Imagine a string through the crown of your head lifting you taller, but at the same time keep the sense of grounding through your feet and legs.

- You can also practise this pose by placing your hands in prayer pose, feeling the chest expand against them.

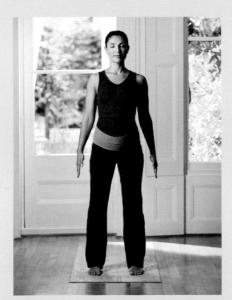 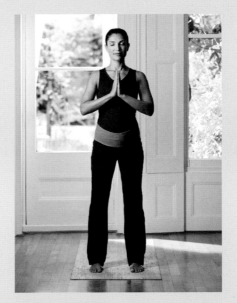

VARIATION

Wide-legged Forward Bend

This exercise is great for strengthening the legs and releasing tension in the shoulders. It calms the mind and can ease backache as it stretches the spine.

1 Stand with your legs wide (about one leg length apart unless you have groin pain) and fold from your hips, bringing your hands to the floor and releasing your head. Feel the stretch down the backs of the legs, but bend the knees if you need to. Avoid bouncing and use your breath to deepen the stretch.

• If you feel too much pressure in your head, just come halfway down, resting your elbows on bent knees, keeping your head facing forward.

• If you feel uncomfortable folding forward, you can practise this stretch standing tall with your hands still clasped behind you. This will also help to open your chest.

2 Interlace your fingers, draw your shoulder blades together and extend your arms over your head. With each exhalation release your arms a little bit farther away from your back.

3 Inhale and as you exhale release your hands farther away.

4 Round up slowly through your back, keeping your chin tucked in toward your chest and your knees bent.

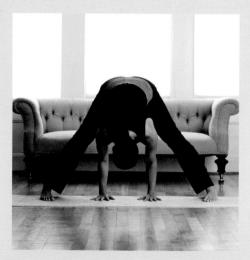

1

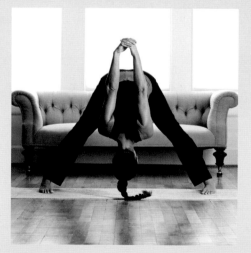

2

Tree

If you are feeling indecisive or "all over the place", this posture can bring focus, balance and clarity to your mind. It also strengthens your legs and ankles and can help with sciatica and flat feet. Avoid if you have groin pain.

1 Find a wall or chair for support if you need it (and turn to one side using your left hand on the support). Shift your weight into your left foot with the foot pointing straight ahead. Press through all the toes and don't let your foot roll.

2 Lift your right leg, placing your foot on your inner thigh (but not against the knee), opening your knee out to the side. Keep your hips facing forward.

3 If you have your balance, place your palms together and raise them high, opening your arms as they extend up into a "V" shape and keeping your shoulders down, away from your ears.

• If you have high blood pressure, you can practise this movement keeping your arms down by your sides or in prayer pose. If balance is a problem, place your foot on your inner calf.

4 Soften your gaze, focus on a point in the distance and keep your breath fluid. PAUSE Hold for as long as you feel comfortable and steady. Aim for 5 slow, relaxed breaths.

5 Gently lower your foot, then repeat Steps 1–4 on the other leg. PAUSE 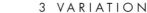 Notice if you feel more balanced on one side. Try to feel an equal stretch on each side of the body.

6 Release your left foot and stand in *Tadasana* (see page 55), feeling the effects of the pose.

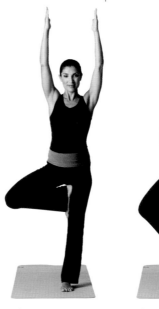

3   3 VARIATION

Warrior

This pose challenges the entire body and helps to open up the chest and lungs while strengthening the arms, back and legs. On an emotional level, it can act as an outward expression of determination and resolve in preparation for labour. Avoid if you have any groin pain.

1 From *Tadasana* (see page 55) step your left leg back 3ft (about 1m), keeping the ball of your foot pressing down and lifting your heel.

2 Reach your arms up toward the ceiling, keeping your shoulders down. Square your hips and lengthen your tailbone toward the floor.

3 Inhaling, lower your left knee to hover just above the floor. At the same time, keep both arms high. Gaze forward and lift through your torso. Aim to stay in this position for 5 breaths.

4 Exhaling, lift your left knee, pressing your arms down with your palms downward. Straighten both legs. Repeat the sequence 3 times, stepping forward with your left leg, then repeat the pose with the other leg forward.

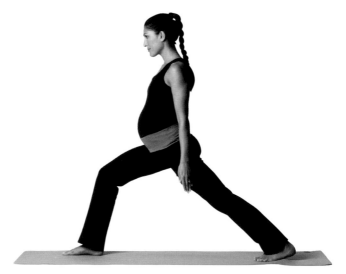

1

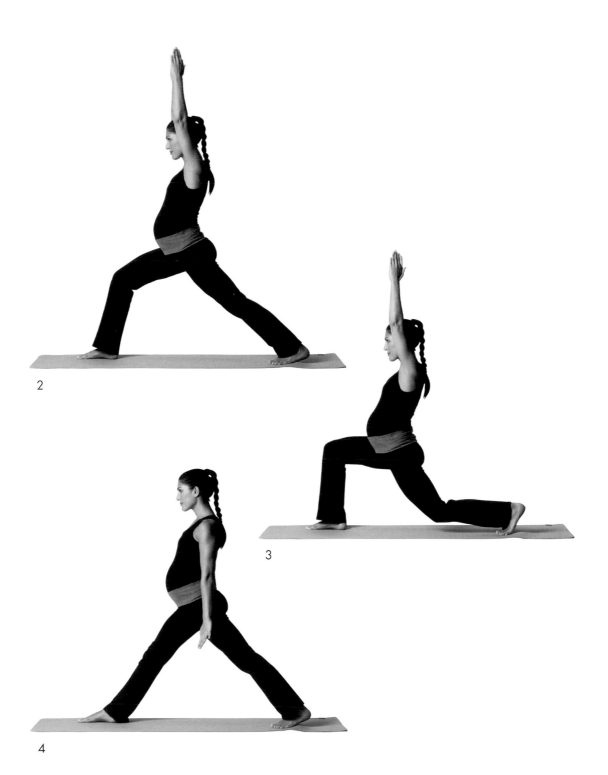

2

3

4

Horse

This is a great pose for opening up the hips and strengthening the legs and inner thigh muscles in preparation for labour. If you would like to have an active birth, it helps to have strong legs so that you can move around and hold a squat position, which can facilitate the second stage of labour by creating more space in the pelvis, harnessing the effects of gravity. Furthermore, developing strength and stamina in your legs throughout pregnancy will help you to feel grounded – not only rooted physically to the earth but, because yoga can give you a deeper sense of yourself, grounded in your life.

The lotus flower *mudra* (hand gesture) that forms part of this pose symbolizes purity and the heart. The fact that a beautiful lotus flower can emerge from the murky depths of a pond is a metaphor for the flowering of new beginnings. Avoid Horse if you have groin pain, or practise the modified version against a wall.

1 Stand with your legs wide, turn your feet out and bend into a squat, keeping your back straight. Let your knees move out toward your toes. As you bend, bring the heels of your hands together and open out your fingers to make the shape of a lotus flower.

- If you have groin pain, keep your feet parallel, using a wall to lean your back against as you come into the squat.

2 Straighten your legs and lift your arms up above your head.

3 Bring the tips of your fingers to touch each other, separating the heels of your hands and pointing your fingers down toward the floor as you bend your knees. Keep the movement as fluid as possible.

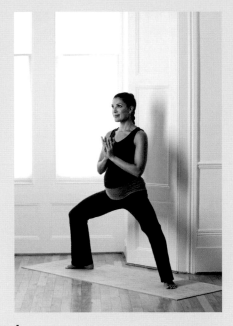

1

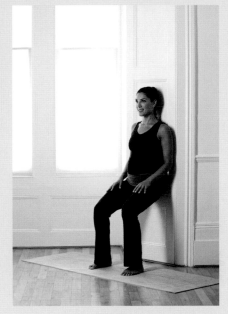

1 VARIATION

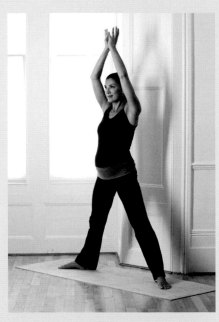

2

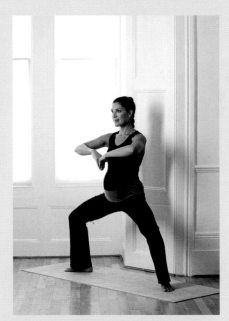

3

Leg Rotations on All Fours

This leg exercise is useful for toning and strengthening your legs and outer thighs, encouraging blood circulation and mobilizing your hip joints. Low-impact activities such as swimming, therapies such as massage, and yoga postures such as the one shown here as well as Pigeon (see page 106), Cow-faced Pose (see page 103), Eagle (see pages 101–102) and various hip-circling exercises (see pages 117, 121 and 122–3) are all helpful for stretching and releasing tension from the hip area. Practise the stretches to prevent tightness building in the hips, which can lead to lower back pain. Avoid this exercise if you are suffering from groin pain. Alternatively, you could modify it by keeping the circles very small.

1 Start on all fours with your weight evenly distributed on each side, your shoulders directly above your wrists and your neck straight so that your head faces down.

2 Lift your left knee off the floor and start to circle your left leg, keeping the knee bent. Extend through the foot so that your leg feels enlivened and energized. Try not to lean to one side – keep the weight evenly spread through both hands. Start with 5 circles and gradually build up the repetitions.

3 Change direction, circling on the same leg. Imagine drawing a circle with your knee and feel the full range of the movement. Keep breathing! If it feels uncomfortable, make the circles smaller.

4 Now change legs, circling one way and then the other as before. Take a rest whenever you need to.

5 Rest in Child's Pose (see pages 80–81) when you have finished.

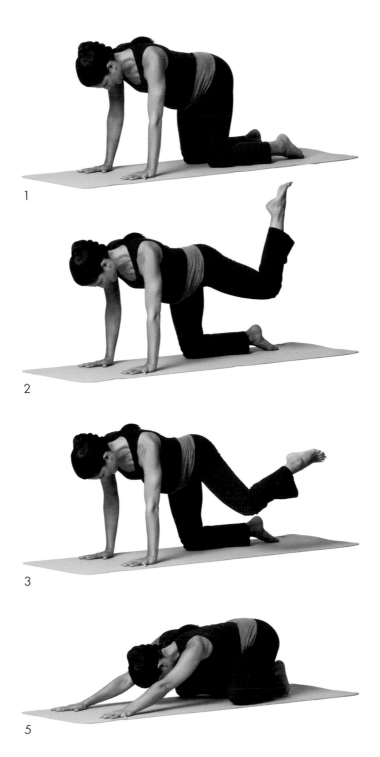

1

2

3

5

Salute to the Sun

The Salute to the Sun is probably one of the best-known yoga *vinyasas* (series of postures linking breath and movement). Traditionally, the sun salutation was practised in the morning, taking the sun's energy into the body, mind and spirit in preparation for the day ahead. It exercises different muscle groups, improves cardiovascular strength and can help to cleanse, tone and revitalize you on every level. It is a good sequence to practise on days when you feel a little lethargic and in need of an energy boost. Over time you will build up your strength, but don't overdo it if you are new to yoga.

As you practise the Salute to the Sun you may like to imagine that you are dancing with your baby through the movements. The rocking back and forth in a lunge can be used during the second stage of labour to help the pelvis present different angles for the baby to emerge into the world.

1 Stand at the front of your mat, feet hip-width apart, palms in prayer pose.

2 As you inhale, raise your arms above your head, keeping them shoulder-width apart.

3 As you exhale, bend your knees and bring your palms down via your heart centre.

4 Continue down until your palms reach the floor in front of your feet and straighten your legs if you can.

5 Inhale and as you exhale step your left foot back into a lunge, keeping your hips low, with your left knee on the floor. Make sure your right knee is above your right ankle.

6 Rest your left knee on the floor and bend your right knee, making sure it doesn't come too far forward. Rest your hands on your front thigh. Lift up through your spine.

7 Inhale, bringing your weight forward toward the front toes.

8 Exhale, shifting the weight back so that your back leg forms a right-angle. Repeat the forward and backward motion 3 times.

9 On an inhale, lift your back knee off the floor, feeling strong through your legs, and keeping your front knee above your ankle.

10 Bring your back knee down to the floor and move your hands to the floor, too. Inhale and tuck the toes of your back foot under.

11 Move your front leg back so you are now kneeling on all fours.

12 As you exhale, lift up through the hips into Downward Dog (avoid this during the last weeks of pregnancy). Press down through your hands and fingers and feel the stretch in your hamstrings as you shift weight back through your hips into your heels. Try not to hunch your shoulders up to your ears.

13 Breathe deeply. As you inhale lift your heels, coming onto the balls of your feet. As you exhale, lower them back down, inhaling as you lift, exhaling as you release. Repeat a few times, feeling a stretch through all the toes.

14 Lower the knees down so that you are back on all fours.

15 As you inhale step your right foot forward into a lunge. If you are finding it difficult to get your foot all the way forward to your hands, you can use one hand to help shuffle it forward. Bring your hands onto your front thigh and rock back and forth, inhaling forward and exhaling back. Feel a stretch through the front thigh and hip. (Do not do this if have groin pain.) Lower your hands back to the floor.

16 Inhaling, step your left foot forward like a frog so that you are now in a standing forward bend. Release your neck, keeping a bend in your knees.

17 Inhale and start to unravel your spine slowly back up, vertebra by vertebra, keeping your chin toward your chest, bringing your head back to the centre.

18 Finally, raise your arms back up, palms touching at your heart centre.

19 Repeat on the other side, this time taking your right leg back. Repeat 3–4 times if you want to challenge yourself and build up your strength and stamina, but make sure that you listen to your body and don't force or over-exert yourself.

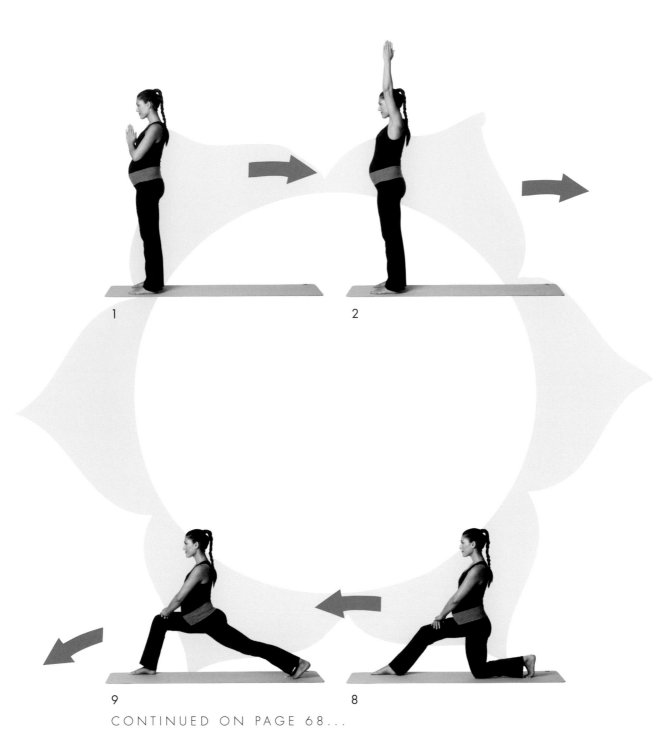

1

2

9

8

CONTINUED ON PAGE 68...

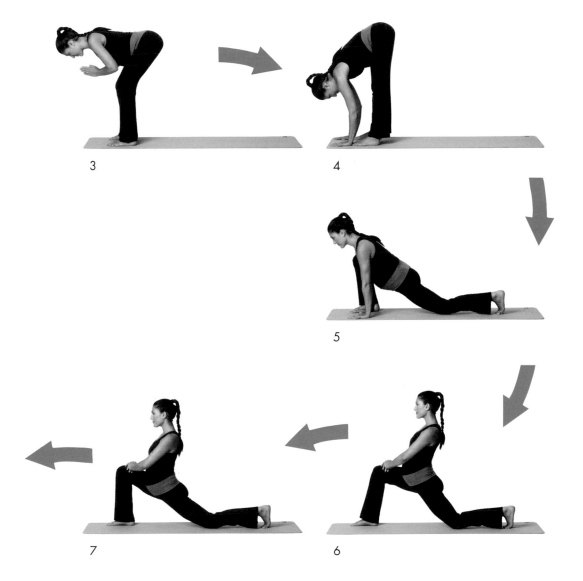

3

4

5

6

7

... CONTINUED FROM PAGE 66

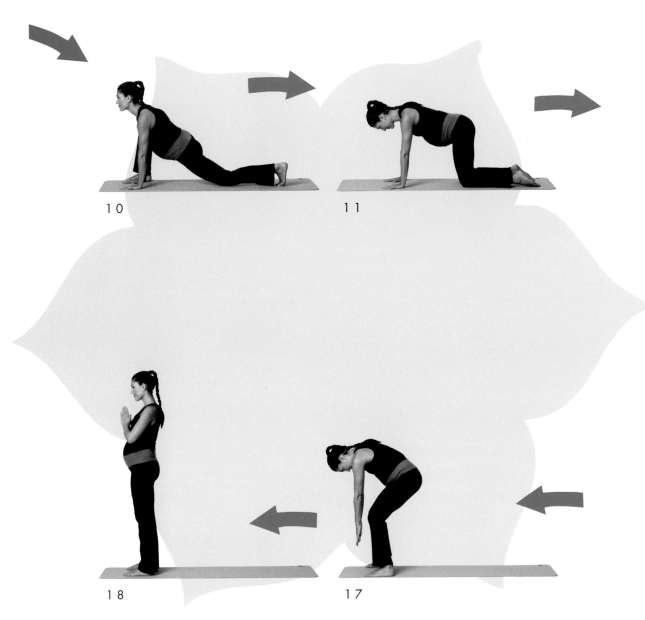

10

11

18

17

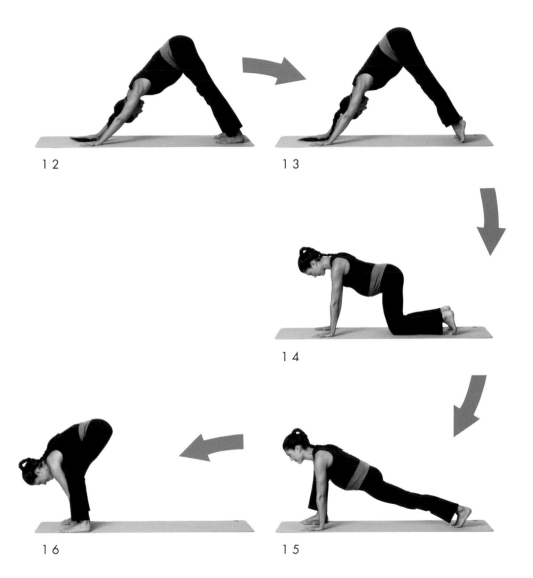

12

13

14

15

16

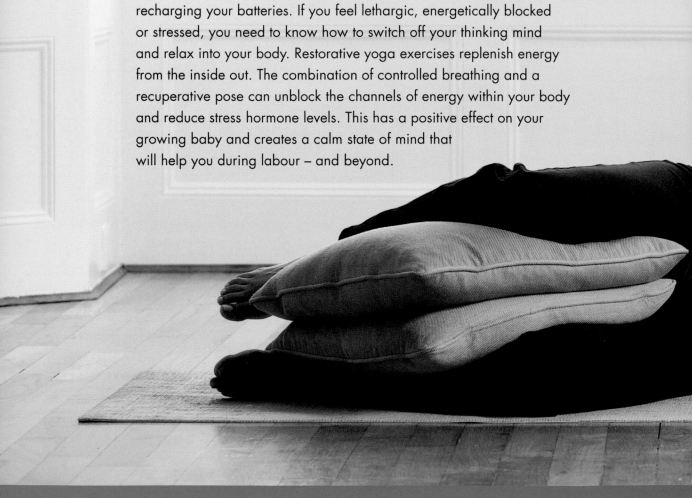

CHAPTER 4
Relax and Restore

Relaxing during pregnancy is very important for releasing tension and recharging your batteries. If you feel lethargic, energetically blocked or stressed, you need to know how to switch off your thinking mind and relax into your body. Restorative yoga exercises replenish energy from the inside out. The combination of controlled breathing and a recuperative pose can unblock the channels of energy within your body and reduce stress hormone levels. This has a positive effect on your growing baby and creates a calm state of mind that will help you during labour – and beyond.

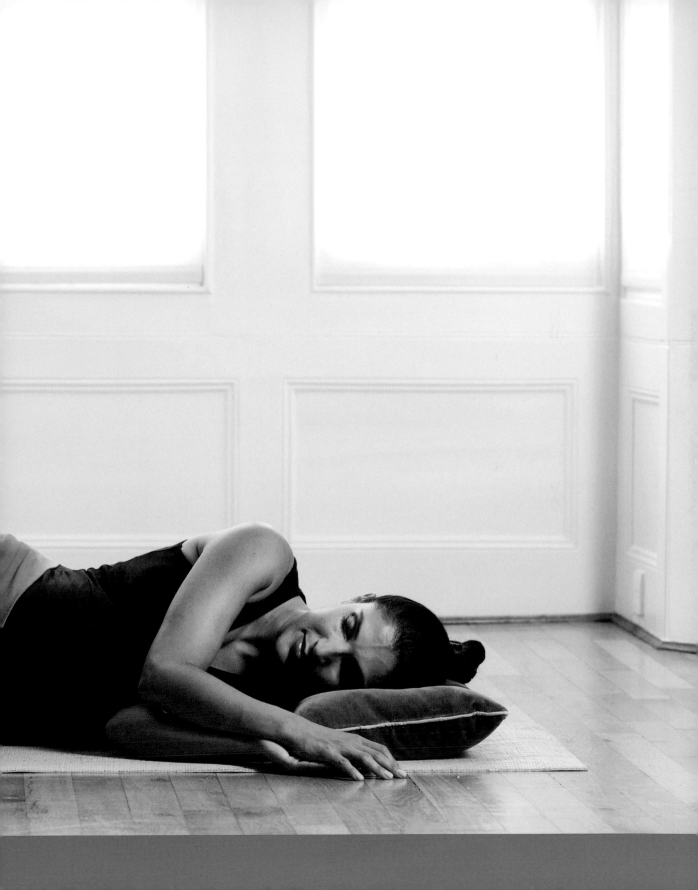

Affirmations

I feel confident and relaxed.

I rest and nurture myself to build my energy levels.

I have reserves of energy that I can
draw on during my labour.

I can let go of anxieties and fears and trust
that my body knows what to do.

I have support from people around me.

I send healing energy and vitality to my baby.

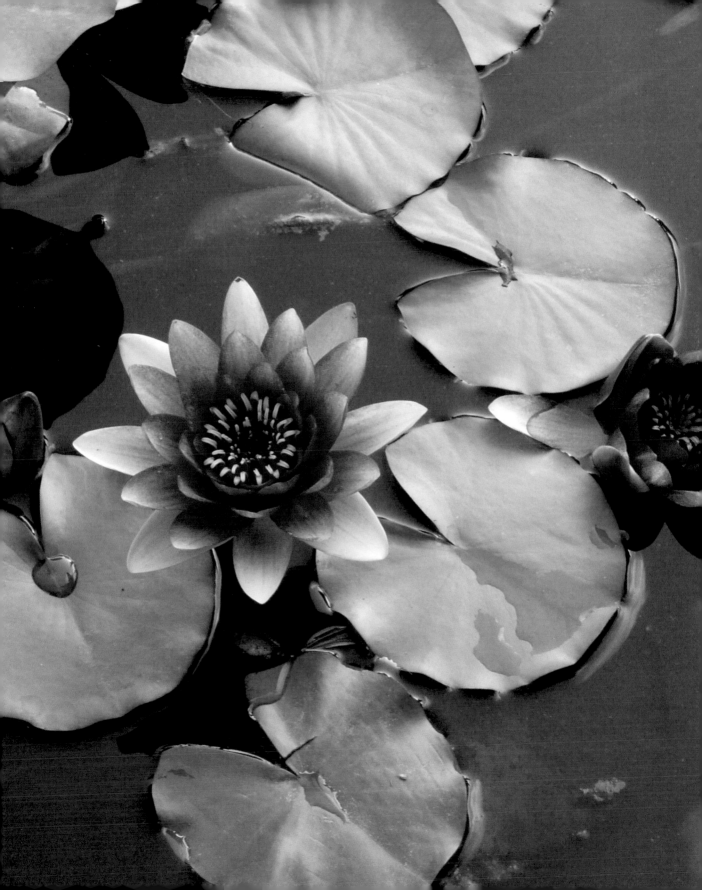

Learning to Let Go

Calm and restful awareness is the most natural human state, but our busy modern lives tend to make us forget this and we become disconnected from our true selves. Rediscovering inner peace while you are pregnant can feel like coming home. Not only do you have a personal sanctuary within, you are also providing a safe place for your baby to grow – practising specific relaxation and restorative poses for the mind and body will have a deeply peaceful effect on you both, bringing you closer to your natural state of intuition, in which you can hear and trust your inner voice. Pregnancy is not just a journey toward the birth of your child but is also a rite of passage into motherhood.

During pregnancy many of us carry a multitude of emotions and some of these may be fearful or anticipatory. This is normal, particularly for first-time mothers. Quietening your mind and letting it achieve a state of relaxation has a similar effect on your body, and vice versa. In other words, practising restorative poses and relaxing your body also calm your mind.

When you are practising yoga it is important to realize that different poses have different energetic effects. Some are stimulating and others make you feel more relaxed according to how you feel on any given day. This also applies to the seasons and the time of day. As you become more in tune with your body you understand which yoga practice – whether a single posture or a sequence, a meditation or a specific breathing exercise – will bring you back into balance.

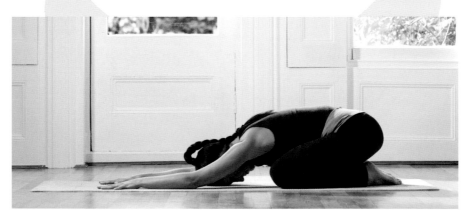

Learning to breathe deeply when facing stressful situations or feeling anxious can help you to dissolve physical and emotional tension. By practising *Savasana* (see pages 84–5) and Child's Pose (see pages 80–81) throughout pregnancy, your body will instinctively enter a state of relaxation when you come into these poses in labour.

And remember ... learn how to nap! This skill will be invaluable in the early months with a newborn.

Birth Story ...

"The most profound effect of restorative yoga was that it enabled me to embrace without fear the prospect of giving birth. Through yoga I learned to listen to my body and trust its capabilities. My first labour was scheduled to be a home birth, but as the labour dragged on and my cervix wouldn't fully dilate, eventually I transferred to hospital and my son was delivered by forceps. But I never felt that the birthing experience was 'taken away' from me. Throughout I was able to stay present – at each juncture accepting what was or wasn't happening – and make the necessary choices to deliver my baby safely. Three years later when I had my daughter it was completely different. Again I planned for a home birth, but this time things moved on a lot more quickly and consequently the experience was much more intense. What saw me through was a complete focus on the breath and on the present moment. The few instances when it nearly felt overwhelming – when my response could have turned into panic – my mind took me beyond thoughts of 'How long will this go on? What if I can't take it any longer?' In those moments, completely committing to coming back to the breath, to riding the surges or contractions one at a time, was what saw me through. My daughter was born at home in our bed and it was amazing to experience this completely natural yet miraculous event. I relied on the physical strength as well as the strength of mind, the focus, that I had built up during my yoga practice." **Tanja**

GETTING COMFORTABLE

Relaxation is as important as the active poses we have explored in previous chapters. This is a time for you to let go completely, allowing the benefits of your yoga practice to integrate with your mind, your body and your baby. Learning how to relax is a great mental preparation for labour, helping you to utilize the pauses between contractions to replenish and restore your energy. Finding a comfortable position in late pregnancy is not always easy, but the following selection of seated and lying positions should be helpful.

Legs on a Chair/Sofa

This is good to do if you are under 25 weeks pregnant (providing you still feel OK to lie on your back) and have tired legs or swollen feet, ankles or legs.

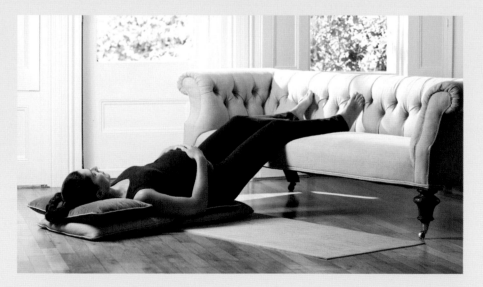

Lie on your back with cushions or a folded blanket for support under your lower back and under your head, and rest with your legs bent on a chair or a sofa. Remain here for as long as you like.

Sitting on a Chair

In late pregnancy, you will increasingly feel the need to sit down to relieve the burden of the extra weight you are carrying. We have already looked at the right and wrong way to sit for yoga practice (see page 34), but you will also benefit from finding the correct position when you are just relaxing.

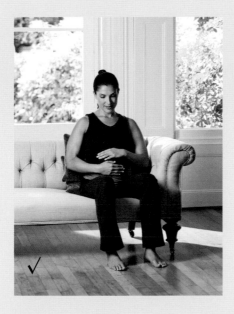

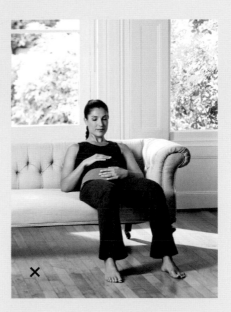

CORRECT
Make sure you sit up tall using a cushion behind your back and under your feet, if required.

INCORRECT
Try to resist the temptation to lean back into a sofa or an armchair. If you slouch, it puts pressure on the back and may also encourage your baby to move into a posterior position. This is something you want to avoid, if possible.

Leaning/Resting on a Chair

Nagging physical discomfort, such as an aching back, can distract the mind and get in the way of relaxation. Bending and stretching using a reasonably high-backed chair or sofa for support is a great way to gently relieve pressure on the back. Sitting "the wrong way round" on a chair is another position that takes weight off the lower spine.

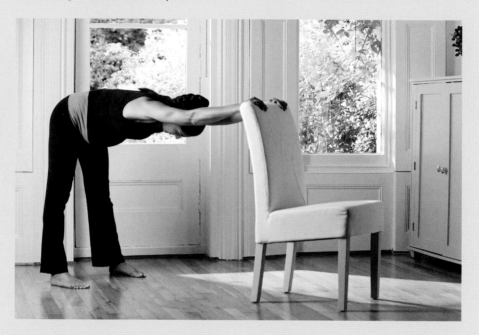

LEANING ON A CHAIR

Find a sturdy chair (or a sofa). If the chair is likely to move, place it next to a wall. Stand with your feet parallel to it – about 3½ft (1m) away – and reach your arms out, resting your hands on top of the chair or sofa back. Try not to collapse into your lower back – keep it as straight as possible. Breathe deeply as you feel your spine lengthening, anchoring down through your heels and moving your hips back. Use this position whenever you feel tightness or pressure in your back. This is a good alternative to Downward Dog (see Salute to the Sun, pages 64–9) if you are in the last few weeks of your pregnancy.

RESTING ON A CHAIR

This is a great position for relaxing or chatting to friends, as it releases pressure from your lower spine and allows your pelvis to tilt, taking the weight of the baby off your spine and encouraging it into the optimal foetal position. Find a chair with no arms, turn it around and sit with one leg on each side, resting one hand lightly on the other arm.

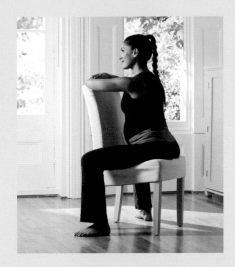

Resting on the Back with Feet Against the Wall

This pose gently relaxes the hamstrings. Tight hamstrings can pull the pelvis and cause back pain.

Lying on your back (if you are under 25 weeks pregnant), using cushions for support, can be a wonderfully relaxing pose in its own right. You can lie with your legs straight and your feet against the wall. Feel the stretch in your hamstrings. Come out of the pose after a few minutes (earlier if you feel any discomfort) by bending your knees toward you, keeping them wide, and rolling onto one side before you sit up.

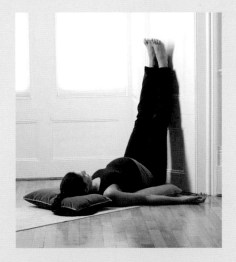

Child's Pose

This is a wonderful restorative pose that is useful for replenishing your energy and releasing tension in between contractions during labour. You can use it whenever you need to rest during pregnancy or if you feel dizzy when you are practising any of the exercises. As this pose is designed for relaxation, it is particularly important that you feel comfortable in it. Use the suggested modifications, if necessary, to make it work for you.

1 On all fours bring your knees wide apart, big toes touching, and sit back on your heels if possible.
- If your sit bones don't reach your heels, place a pillow there (see below).
- If you have groin pain, keep your knees closer together and stay upright closing your eyes.

2 Extend your arms forward to lengthen your spine.
- If you prefer to keep your head up, cup your chin in your hands (see opposite).

- If you are not comfortable on the floor or your bump is big, you can raise your arms on cushions and make a pillow with your hands, turning your head to one side (see opposite).

3 Soften your face, relax your jaw and breathe deeply (releasing the jaw is linked to softening the cervix). Think about breathing into your back and let go. Focus on your breath, and whenever your mind wanders bring your attention back to your breathing.

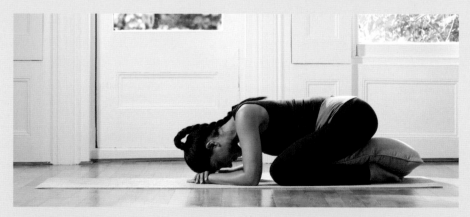

1 VARIATION A

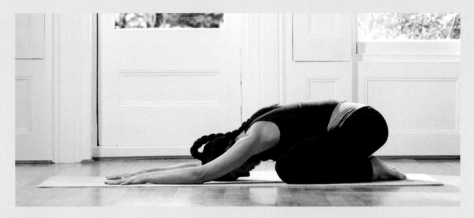

2

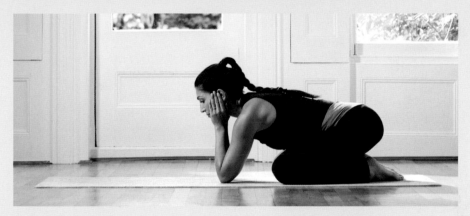

2 VARIATION A

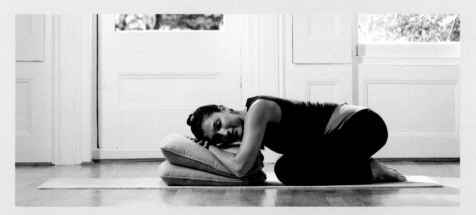

2 VARIATION B

Goddess Meditation

This powerful meditation celebrates motherhood and the creation of new life. It ends with an affirmation giving the meaning of *namaste*, a Sanskrit word used throughout the Indian sub-continent as a salutation and usually accompanied by a prayer gesture that represents the divine spark within each of us.

1 Sit cross-legged and rest your hands on your baby in *yoni mudra.* Your fingers point down toward your pelvis and the tips of the thumbs touch, as do the index fingers, making a womb shape.

2 Focus on the rise and fall of your baby being massaged with each breath. Breathe deeply and start to bring your awareness deeper inside your body. Visualize your baby safe and sound in your womb. PAUSE ❀ See yourself as a beautiful, powerful woman, a creator of life, a spiritual being. Feel honoured that you are able to nurture this new life within you. Marvel at the power that you have been given. Celebrate your body growing new life; be awed at your blooming fuller form; see yourself as a source of creation at its most inspiring … You are part of an incredible, unique process in which, miraculously, your body knows exactly what to do. You are a Goddess … Tune into how this feels and what it means to you. You are staying centred and grounded as you progress through each stage of this wonderful and exciting journey into motherhood. Take this amazing opportunity that you are fortunate to have and build your sense of inner power … you, too, are a miracle of creation. Allow yourself to be a light shining for others. Be all that you can be. Feel courageous and empowered. Honour the Goddess within you. Feel gratitude for what you are experiencing. Your life will change forever once you welcome your baby into the world and hold it in your arms. You feel more love for this precious being, this sacred gift, than you ever thought possible.

3 Start to come back to the sensation of your breath moving in your abdomen. Rub your hands together in front of your heart until they feel warm. Place one hand on top of the other over your heart. Feel the warmth from your hands

and imagine it radiating throughout your body, sealing the energy and intention from this meditation deep within you. Now, placing one hand on your baby, and keeping the other hand on your heart, connect with your baby, sending it joy, courage, love and strength.

4 Finally, bow your chin toward your heart. If you wish, turn your hands upward, pressing your palms and fingers together in front of your chest in the *namaste* gesture. Give thanks as you honour the life growing within you: "I honour the place where the entire universe resides. I honour the feeling of truth, love, light and peace. I honour the feeling where, if you are in that place in you and I am in that place in me, there is only one of us."
Namaste

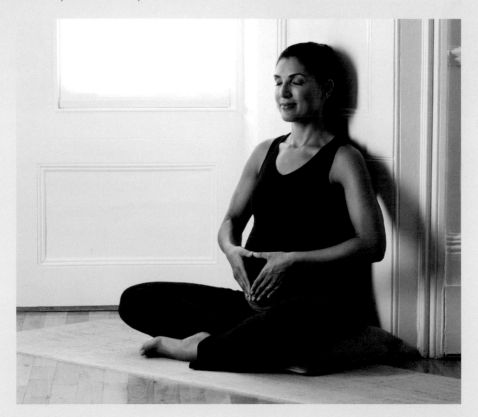

Savasana

As already mentioned, it is advisable to avoid lying on your back in the last months of pregnancy as this can put pressure on your spine and may restrict blood flow, making you feel dizzy and nauseous. If you are in your last trimester, or feel uncomfortable on your back, lie on your left side instead – this encourages your baby into the optimum position for birth and assists your heart and blood flow. Placing a cushion (or cushions) either under your right leg or between both legs will take pressure off your pelvis. Cushions underneath your knees will release your lower back, and for comfort you can place a cushion under your head, too (see Variations A and B, opposite). Close your eyes and rest here, enjoying the feeling of being supported.

1 Relax … let go. Soften your eyes and all the little muscles around your eyes, release your jaw, relax the root of your tongue and let it rest on the roof of your mouth. Release the base of your skull, soften across your forehead and top of your head, soften your neck and relax your throat, your centre of creativity, change and expression, which is heightened during pregnancy. Release your shoulders away from your ears and visualize sending any stress and tension down your arms and out through your fingers. Soften the front of your body, relax your chest and release deep into your abdomen, sending this sense of peace to your growing baby. Relax the back of your body, releasing your upper back, softening the middle of your back and relaxing the lower back all the way down to your sacrum. Release your pelvis, softening your hips and buttocks and relax all the way down through your legs to your feet and toes. Imagine that your body is melting into the floor and see if you can let go even more now. Gently bring your awareness to your breathing, clearing your mind of any thoughts for the last minute or so. PAUSE Remain here with your mind free of thought for a minute or longer. Any time a thought arises, gently bring your focus back to your breath.

2 Now imagine a golden light spreading from your navel in all directions, bringing energy to every single cell,

every muscle and every organ of your body. With each breath, this golden light becomes stronger and stronger, permeating through your whole body, healing any areas that need healing. See the golden light circling and enveloping your baby with protection, sending energy to your baby for its growth and development. Imagine that this light is connecting your heart to your baby's heart and send love to your baby. PAUSE 🪷 Thank yourself for taking the time out to do your yoga, remembering that by nurturing yourself you are also nurturing your baby.

3 Stay here for as long as you want – you may find that you fall asleep. To come out of this relaxation, make sure that you come up slowly, taking time to sit and tune in to any sensations within your body and your mind.

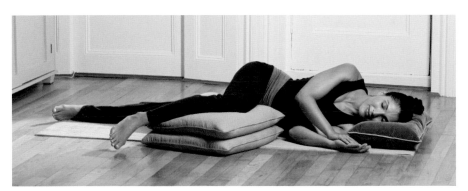

LYING VARIATION A

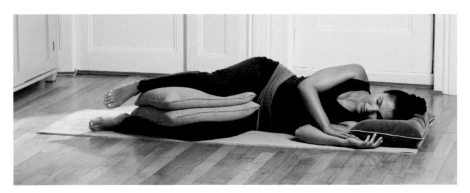

LYING VARIATION B

CHAPTER 5
Common Ailments and Conditions

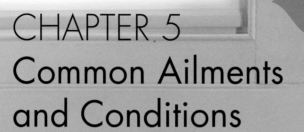

Throughout pregnancy your body and your mind will undergo immense changes. Yoga is one of the best ways of managing the additional demands put upon your body, of easing discomfort and of coping with the ups and downs of your emotional state. Knowing that you have yoga at your disposal to alleviate the symptoms of pregnancy-related ailments will feel incredibly empowering.

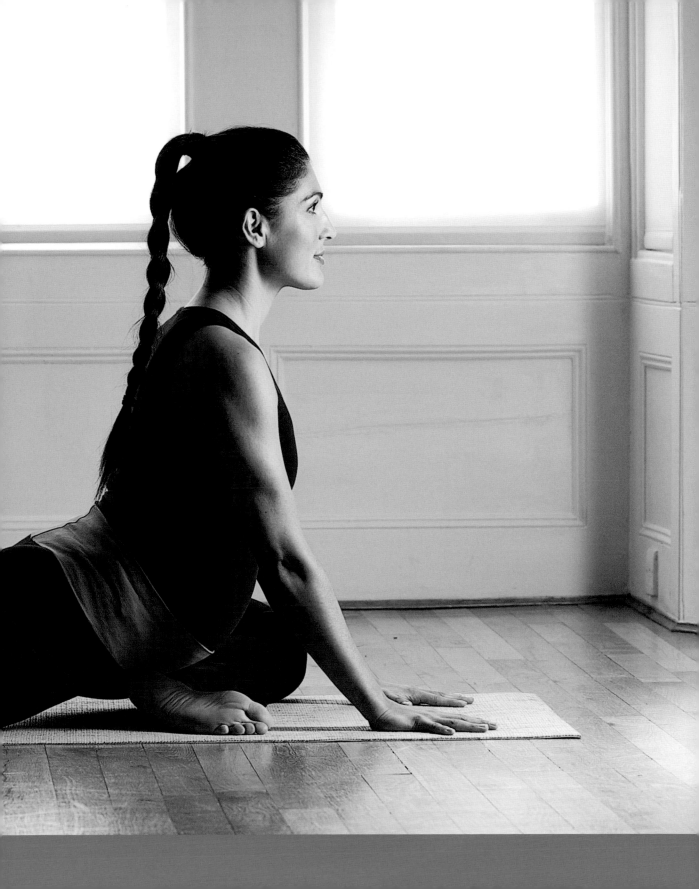

Affirmations

I send healing energy and light to the
places where I feel discomfort.

I notice how my body feels without judging or
becoming fixed on any uncomfortable sensations.

I realize that uncomfortable feelings are
temporary and will pass over time.

I accept and welcome the changes in my body
that each stage of pregnancy brings.

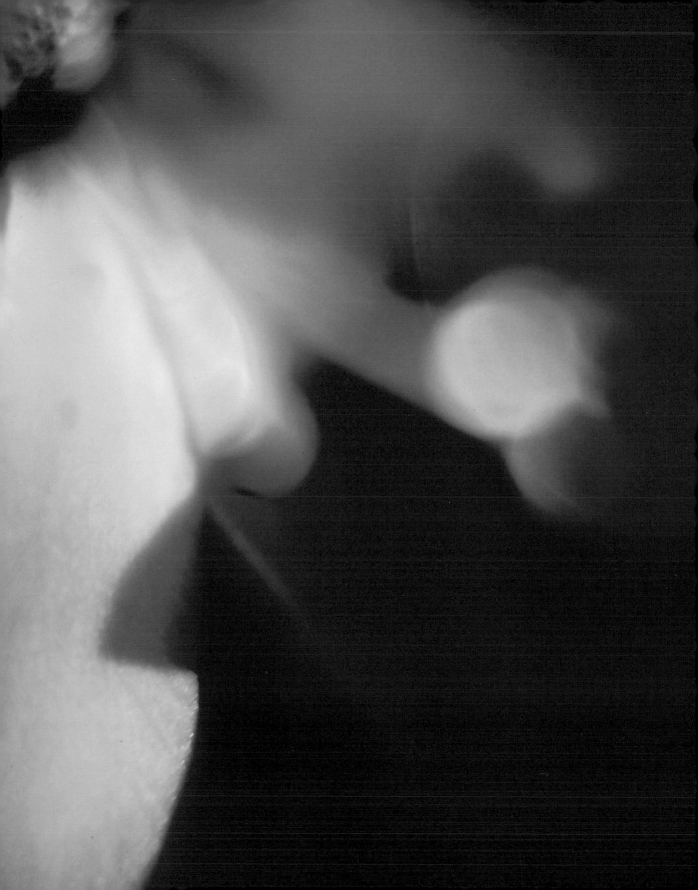

Looking after Yourself

Pregnancy should be about being in a state of health, and not about suffering. The notion of a woman eating for two and becoming increasingly immobile and awkward as her baby grows has become outdated. This does not mean you should put yourself under pressure to be a "supermum" and place unrealistic demands on yourself. It is important to find the right balance of activity and rest and to nourish yourself without over-indulging. Yoga brings equilibrium in both mind and body. The postures recommended in this chapter not only help to relieve pregnancy-related symptoms, but they also work on the brain to balance your emotional state.

Yoga can help you to accept and interpret the changes that you are going through. Respecting your body, eating wisely and practising yoga during your pregnancy all help to build awareness so you will notice when you are out of balance and can take remedial action. As you move with awareness of the breath, you keep *prana* or energy flowing freely in the channels (*nadis*) of your body, restoring equilibrium and even helping to prevent common ailments from developing in the first place. Many women who regularly do yoga sail through their pregnancy without any problems.

During the first three months (first trimester) the most common symptoms you may experience are fatigue and morning sickness. Many women have heightened emotions and greater sensitivity at all levels – for example, the sense of smell is enhanced and you may experience food cravings. The most common craving is for carbohydrates such as bread, cereals and pasta, rather than meat, fish or eggs, which are more likely to contain harmful bacteria. This is nature's way of protecting your baby at a crucial stage of development. Carbohydrates contain a lot of calories and therefore provide much-needed energy as your baby's spine, brain and organs develop.

Physically challenging yoga postures are not advisable until after your first scan (usually at 12–14 weeks) on account of the huge changes that are taking place and because the risk of miscarriage is higher until this time. So go easy during this period and take a rest when your body needs it.

Apart from visible changes, such as your breasts and your bump getting bigger, there are many invisible changes going on inside you. For example, your oestrogen levels rise dramatically, your ovaries enlarge, you produce more blood, and your output of the hormone relaxin increases to help soften all your ligaments ready for birth. This is one reason why during pregnancy you have to take care not to overstretch. Always listen to your body and do what feels right for you.

The exercises in this chapter can help with the most common pregnancy ailments, but are not intended as a substitute for medical advice. If you have any serious pregnancy-related issues, make sure you consult your doctor first.

You may also want to consider seeing an alternative health practitioner, such as a massage therapist, chiropractor, physiotherapist, acupuncturist, homeopath, osteopath or nutritionist, all of whom may be able to alleviate certain aches and pains. Don't suffer discomfort or wait for it to go away by itself. Go and see a professional if you are at all concerned.

Birth Story ...

"The only thing that made me depressed during my pregnancy was the knowledge that Tara's yoga class would have to come to an end when I gave birth! I really couldn't recommend it more. It had the brilliant balance of being dynamic as well as deeply relaxing and contemplative. It definitely helped me with the earlier signs of sciatica and I left each class feeling physically and mentally strengthened."
Laura

BACKACHE

The health of your spine is crucial to your overall health as it holds all the pathways of energy to the rest of your body. Many women experience some form of backache during their pregnancy, but beginning yoga at an early stage will reduce the chance of developing it.

Rounding and Straightening

Exercises like this one can release tension in your spine if your back is aching as a result of carrying extra weight from your baby in the front of your body.

1 Bring your feet onto the floor in front of you with your knees bent. Place your hands on your knees or shins and, as you inhale, draw your shoulders back and press against your shins to lift up and extend taller through your spine.

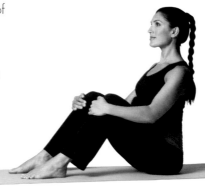

2 As you exhale, drop your chin toward the chest and round through your back and shoulders, releasing tension.

1

3 Keep synchronizing your breath with your movement – inhaling, feeling your lungs expanding; exhaling, sinking back through the pelvis and softening. Do this at your own pace for 5–10 rounds.

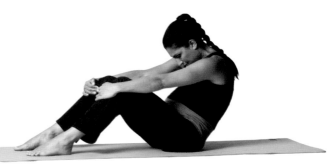

2

Opposite Arm and Leg Raises

This exercise really helps to strengthen your lower back and will improve your balance. It is a good one to do after Cat and Swooping Cat (see pages 48–9), which assists flexibility and blood flow to the spine.

1 Kneel on all fours with your knees directly under your hips.

2 As you inhale, extend your right arm in front and your left leg behind, no higher than your hip. PAUSE 🪷 Keep your gaze down. Check that your hips are in line, that your supporting arm is firm and that you are not locking your elbow or hyper-extending.

3 Exhale, lower to all fours, and on the inhale lift your opposite arm and leg. Feel strong and stable as you move with each breath.

4 Inhale, stretching through your back, lengthening from your fingers through to your toes. If you feel any discomfort in your lower back, extend the leg back but do not lift it off the floor.

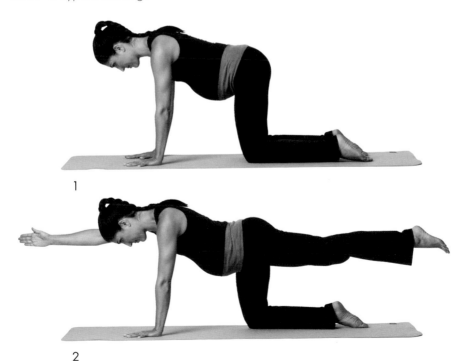

1

2

BREATHLESSNESS

You may experience breathlessness as your uterus grows and pushes against the diaphragm and other internal organs. It can also be caused by a high level of progesterone, which tells the brain to lower carbon dioxide (CO_2) levels in the blood. This results in faster and deeper breathing to exhale more CO_2. Breathlessness can be a symptom of iron deficiency (especially when coupled with fatigue). Always check your symptoms with a doctor. The exercises in Chapters 1 and 2 are also helpful.

Elbow Circles

This exercise opens up the chest, improving lung capacity. It can loosen tight shoulders and improve posture, which also assists breathing.

Sit tall, bring your fingertips to your shoulders and make five big elbow circles in each direction. Keep your shoulders down and relaxed.

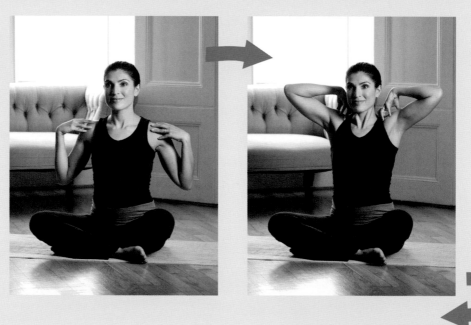

MORNING SICKNESS AND NAUSEA

Pregnancy sickness is generally believed to be caused by an increase in hormones passing through the liver. It is usually helped by eating small snacks to keep levels of blood sugar balanced. Vitamin B_6 is also thought to be effective as it supports liver metabolism. Ginger is another option for relieving nausea, and many women find acupuncture helpful. For most women, the sickness subsides by 12–16 weeks, but unfortunately a small percentage of women feel sick throughout pregnancy.

Lengthening the Breath

This simple breathing exercise is a great way to relieve both breathlessness (see opposite) and nausea. Notice over time if your breathing becomes easier.

Sitting comfortably on the floor, with your legs crossed (or supported by cushions), and your hands resting on your baby, start to slow down and lengthen your breath. Close your eyes. As you inhale through your nose, count 4 in your mind: 1, 2, 3, 4, and then exhale: 1, 2, 3, 4. Keep your eyes closed and repeat. If 4 counts aren't possible, see if you can build up gradually. If you want to lengthen your breath further, add 1–2 more counts. Count slowly. Try not to force the breath – keep it smooth, fluid and consistent.

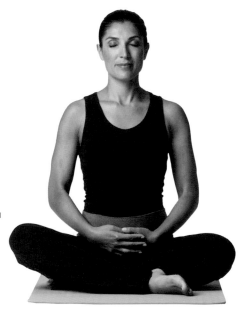

BREECH BABY

If your baby is in a breech presentation, there are a number of strategies you can use to help it find the optimal position for birthing. You can try your best, but don't feel dejected if your baby doesn't oblige – it may just be more comfortable in the position it has chosen! If your baby hasn't turned by 37 weeks, it is less likely to do so because of its size. However, there have been stories of babies turning at the last minute on the way to the operating theatre for a caesarean!

- Acupuncture and moxibustion have a high success rate (over 70 percent in many studies) in helping to turn breech babies.
- Shining a torch and playing music – This may sound like an "old wives' tale", but some of my students have found it works! Shine a torch near the base of your abdomen and your baby will notice the light and may start to move toward it. You can also try playing music, placing the speaker near the base of your abdomen in order to tempt your baby to move in this direction.
- Frozen peas – Placing a bag of frozen peas at the top of your abdomen may encourage your baby to move away from the cold and therefore help it to turn!
- Crawling on all fours – This allows the weight of the baby to move out of the pelvis and into the front of the body, thereby giving your baby more room to move and turn. You can do this whenever you have time or feel like scrubbing the kitchen floor!
- External cephalic version (ECV) – You could ask your doctor about an ECV, a procedure involving gently manipulating your abdomen to turn your baby.
- Visualization – You could also try visualizing your baby in the optimal position (head down with its back facing forward, chin tucked into its chest, preparing for its exit into the world).

On Hands and Knees with Hips High

As well as the strategies discussed opposite, there are various yoga positions that can help to persuade your baby to assume the optimal foetal position.

Move onto your hands and knees and rest your forehead on your forearms. Keep your knees hip-width apart and raise your hips high. Breathe deeply and relax in this position for 5–20 minutes – you can relax here in quiet contemplation or listen to music or a visualization CD.

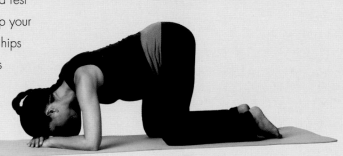

Raising Hips

This pose is another good way to reposition a breech baby.

Lie with your feet on the floor and rest your hips on cushions. This tips your baby out of the pelvis, allowing it more room to move.

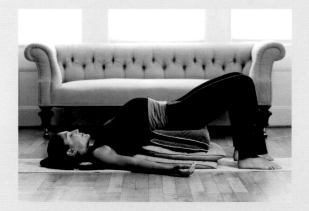

CARPAL TUNNEL SYNDROME

Normally associated with people whose jobs involve repetitive hand movements, such as keyboard operators or factory machinists, carpal tunnel syndrome is also common during pregnancy. This is because fluid retention builds up pressure on the median nerve in the wrist. This nerve supplies feeling and movement to the hand and when restricted can cause numbness, tingling and in some cases intense pain. The symptoms generally subside after childbirth as fluid levels return to normal. During pregnancy there are various ways of relieving the discomfort, such as wearing a wrist splint or practising the following exercise.

Wrist Exercise

This exercise can help to improve circulation to the wrists and hands, and will also strengthen your arms.

1 Inhaling, bring your arms to the front with wrists straight and knuckles down.

2 Exhaling, rotate your arms up, with your wrists bent and knuckles up.

3 Inhaling, open your arms out to your sides to shoulder height.

4 Exhaling, bend your elbows, and bring your fists past your upper ribs.

5 Straighten your arms and extend them behind you.

6 Bring your arms out in front of you again and repeat this sequence 10–20 times, moving with the breath. Notice how concentrating on your breathing helps you to stay focused as your arms get tired and you want to give up. This is a good point to remember for labour!

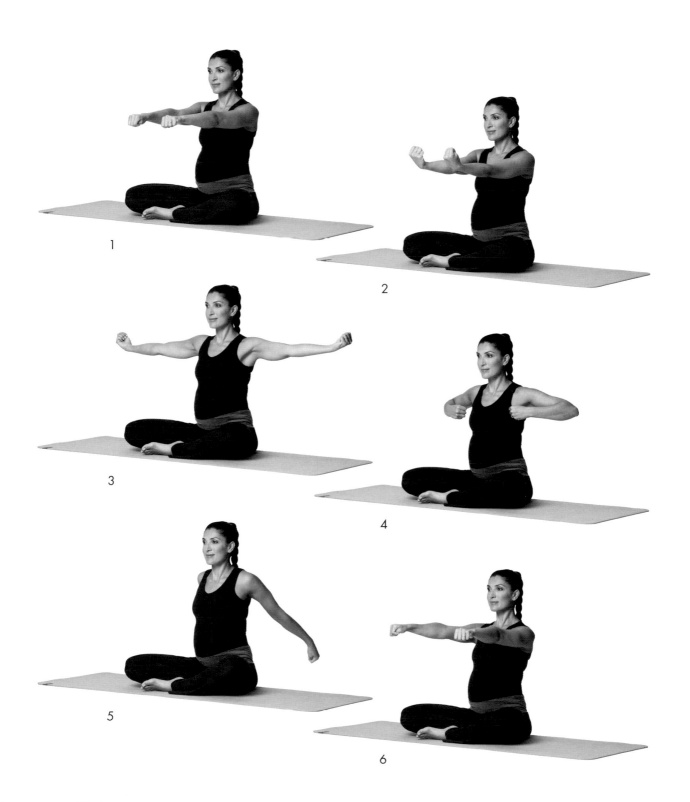

1

2

3

4

5

6

GROIN PAIN AND SYMPHYSIS PUBIS DYSFUNCTION

Groin pain is fairly common in pregnancy and can be severe. It is often caused by the hormone relaxin softening the ligaments, tendons and muscles that support the joints, and it usually occurs any time from the middle of pregnancy onward.

Symphysis pubis dysfunction (SPD) is a condition caused by the relaxing of the ligaments supporting the symphysis pubis joint in order to facilitate birth.

If the ligaments are too loose, the joint becomes unstable and it will probably feel painful to part your legs or to make asymmetrical movements. A related condition is when the gap in the pubic joint widens too much (diastasis symphysis pubis).

Strengthening the lower back and pelvic floor muscles will help to support the groin and pubic area. Take smaller steps when walking, keeping your feet parallel, and try to avoid breaststroke if swimming – just flutter or kick your legs up and down instead. In your yoga practice, avoid any wide-legged yoga poses such as Warrior, *Baddha Konasana*, Horse and seated or standing Wide-legged Forward Bends.

Placing a pillow between your knees whenever you lie down (see page 85) can help to alleviate groin pain and SPD. The pillow will act as a support for the joints around your pelvis and hips, and take away pressure. Practising the following exercises can help to prevent groin pain and SPD, and reduce symptoms if they have already developed.

Eagle

This pose can help to ease groin pain as it draws the muscles and ligaments back in, rather than stretching and opening them. It may also be helpful for sciatica (see page 106), as it releases the hips. With practice your balance should improve and your legs will strengthen. (In addition, the upper body element of the posture relieves tension in the shoulders and upper back, which may be particularly helpful if you spend a lot of time sitting at a desk operating a keyboard.)

1 From a standing position with arms by your sides, bend your knees slightly.

2 Lift your right knee high and wrap your right leg over the left, trying to bring your toes behind your left calf (don't worry if you don't manage to wrap the toes all the way round). Cross your arms and check your balance.

- If you find it difficult to get your balance, you can rest one hand on a wall for support or have your back supported by leaning against a wall.

3 If you feel stable, wrap your right arm over your left, bringing your palms together in line with your nose, and sink a little deeper by bending your supporting leg. Feel the strength in your lower body growing.

- If you find this difficult, you can simply bring your hands into prayer pose (or hold the wall, if you are leaning against one for support).

4 Breathe deeply into this posture, enjoying the feeling of release across your upper back, creating space between your shoulder blades.

5 Stay for 5 breaths, then come out of the pose by pressing your standing foot into the floor to straighten your leg and releasing the intertwined arms and wrapped legs.

6 Now change sides, wrapping your left leg over the right leg and your left arm over the right arm. Stay for 5 breaths, then gently release as before.

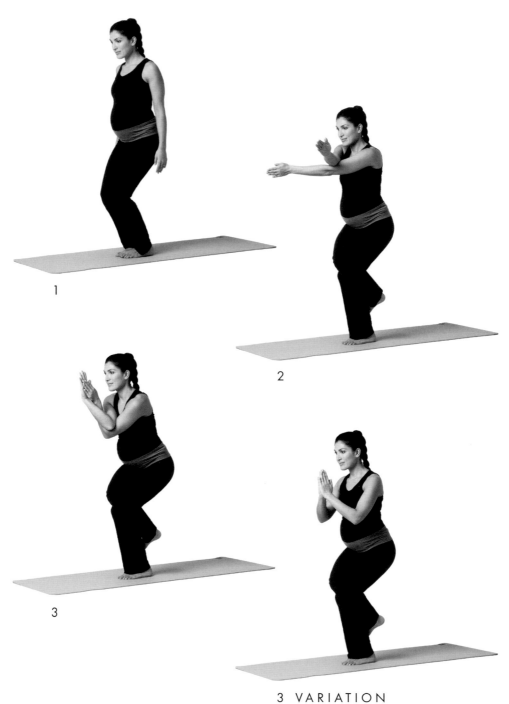

1

2

3

3 VARIATION

Cow-faced Pose

This pose gets its name because your body comes into a shape that resembles the face of a cow, symbolizing a combination of strength and docility. Avoid if you have varicose veins or swollen ankles.

1 Cross your left leg over your right with your knees stacked and feet in line with one another. Sit on the floor with your feet equidistant from your hips if possible. (If you wish, you can sit on blocks or cushions or just cross your legs.) Raise your left arm, pressing your elbow down, and walk your fingers down your back.

2 Bend your right arm (palm facing away) and see whether you can meet your fingers behind your back. PAUSE
✿ Hold the stretch for 5 breaths if possible, breathing deeply into the upper body, bringing the elbows toward the midline, and keeping the head and neck in line. You should feel a strong stretch across your chest, shoulders and triceps (the muscle at the back of the upper arm).

• You can use a strap if your fingers don't touch – take a strap or a belt in your top hand and use it to climb your hands closer toward each other.

3 Change the cross of your legs and repeat on the other side.

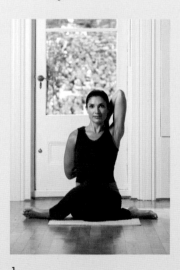 1

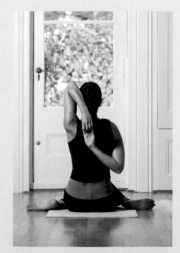 2

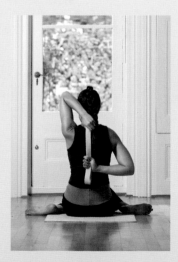 2 VARIATION

HEARTBURN

Heartburn can occur during pregnancy because the muscles of the oesophagus and stomach soften, slowing down digestion and relaxing the valve at the base of the oesophagus. This allows the contents of the stomach to flow back up the oesophagus more easily. As your baby grows bigger the uterus presses against the stomach, making heartburn even more likely.

Yoga helps you to maintain good posture and creates more space in the torso, thereby improving digestive health. Other remedies for heartburn include avoiding large meals, and eating little and often instead. Try not to drink too much liquid with your meals as this dilutes the digestive enzymes. You could also try taking digestive enzyme supplements with your meals.

Leaning Back into Hands

This posture and the wall stretches in Chapter 2 (see page 40) are effective in creating more space for you and your baby, and are particularly beneficial if you are sitting down all day or suffer from indigestion or heartburn.

1 Start in a kneeling position.

2 Place your hands behind you, with fingertips facing forward.

3 Lean back into your hands, lifting your hips away from your heels, opening up through your chest. PAUSE ✦ Hold this position for 3–5 breaths.

4 If you can, release your head back, and allow your chest to open and expand. Breathe into this space with some deep breaths. If you find your head is crunching into your shoulders, keep looking forward.

5 Keep breathing deeply and imagine a thread lifting your sternum up to the sky. Feel your chest expand and release, opening and letting go. As you inhale look forward and, exhaling, release the hips back down. Push into your hands to come back to upright kneeling position.

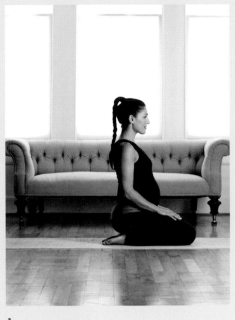

1

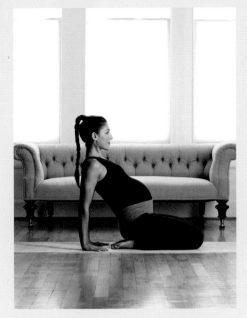

2

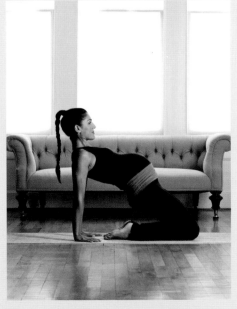

3

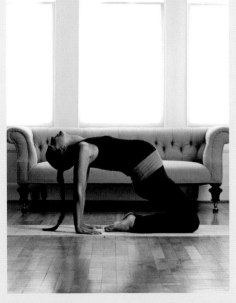

4

SCIATICA

Sciatica can show itself by a shooting pain down the middle of the leg or pain in the centre of the buttocks. In pregnancy it can be caused by the uterus putting pressure on the sciatic nerve. Gentle stretching often helps this condition.

Pigeon

This pose can be practised every day to relieve sciatic pain. It is also great as a general stretch for the muscles round your hips, helping to release emotional and physical tension, which is stored in this area.

1 Place your hands on the floor underneath your shoulders and bring your right knee forward. Try to move your foot farther forward without straining and without rolling onto one side of your hips. Extend your back leg directly behind you with your knee resting on the floor and your toes feeling relaxed.

2 If you are flexible, go forward onto your elbows. PAUSE Breathe deeply into this strong stretch – you should not feel any pain in your knee.

3 Come slowly back up onto all fours and change sides. PAUSE With your mind's eye breathe into your hips and every time you exhale, let go.

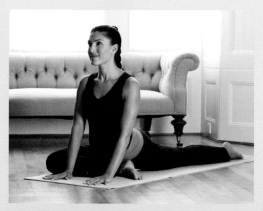

1

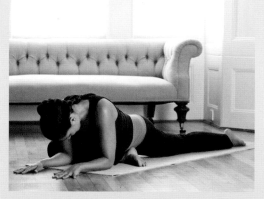

2

LOWER LEG PROBLEMS

Swollen ankles and feet are very common during pregnancy. Your body retains fluid to supply your need for extra blood and to replenish amniotic fluid. Varicose veins may also occur as the expanding uterus puts pressure on the pelvic veins, making it harder for blood to return to the heart from the legs. With more blood circulating and the effect of progesterone relaxing the blood vessels, these may bulge. Avoid sitting, standing or kneeling for long periods. Support socks or tights may be helpful. Many women also find acupuncture helps.

Calf Stretches

Pregnant women are prone to leg cramps, which can be a sign of low potassium levels. Try drinking coconut water or eating bananas to boost your intake of this important mineral. Stretches like this one can also help.

Come onto all fours and stretch one leg back, pressing into the toes and pushing back through the heel. Keep your head looking toward your hands, and your arms straight (without locking the elbows), and breathe here for 3–5 breaths. Push down through your hands as you push through your heel. Breathe deeply for 5–10 breaths. Now change legs and repeat.

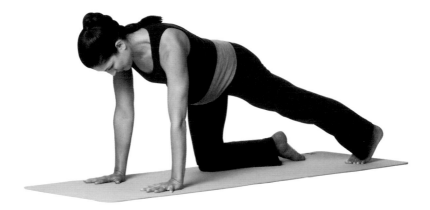

Heel Raises against the Wall and Feet against the Wall

Many women find that their arches collapse during pregnancy – practising these heel raises will help to avoid developing flat feet, as well as strengthening the ankles, which improves balance. Resting your feet against the wall can relieve swollen ankles and feet and varicose veins in the legs.

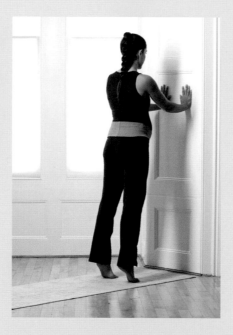 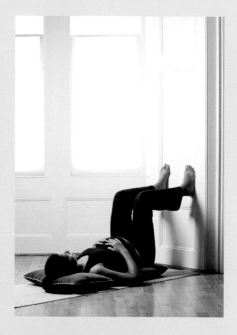

HEEL RAISES AGAINST THE WALL
Stand facing a wall, about 1½ft (40cm) away. Place your palms against the wall, inhale and lift your heels; then exhale and lower them. Raise and lower your heels as many times as feels comfortable, aiming for 5–10 repetitions.

FEET AGAINST THE WALL
If you suffer from varicose veins, simply lying with your feet up against the wall, with bent knees (see above) or legs straight (see page 79), will improve blood flow away from your legs, as well as reducing swelling. Rest on cushions if this is more comfortable.

Foot Circling

Foot circling relieves fluid retention and helps to pump blood back up the legs cleansing the lymphatic system.

1 Stretch your legs in front of you, with feet hip-width apart. Place your hands behind you, with fingers facing you, to keep your back as straight as possible. Circle both feet inward, rotating your ankles. Make 5 big circles.

2 Now change the direction of the circles. Try not to hunch your back as you need to create more space for you and your growing baby.

3 Flex and point your feet alternately and really feel the extension from your heel through to the end of your toes. You should feel a good stretch through your calves. To increase the stretch, lift the heel off the floor as you flex the foot.

4 Now move your feet from side to side keeping your legs loose.

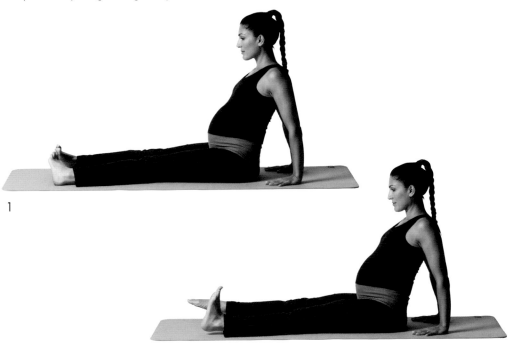

1

3

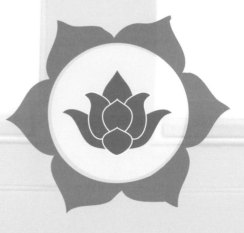

CHAPTER 6
Labour and Childbirth

With all its strengthening and grounding qualities, yoga will help you to feel supported physically and emotionally during your labour and birth experience. It is a good idea to practise the exercises in this chapter throughout your pregnancy so that you are familiar with them before you go into labour. If you are well prepared, you will feel confident that your body knows what to do. Trust this wisdom to guide you through the birth.

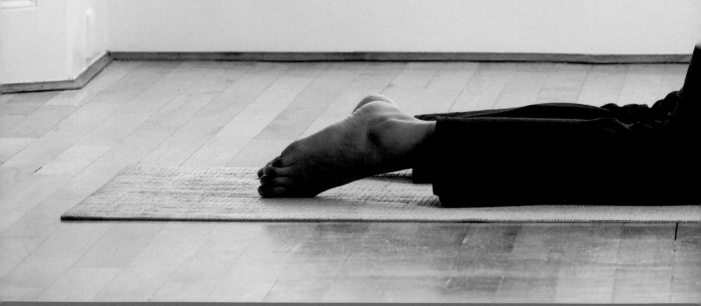

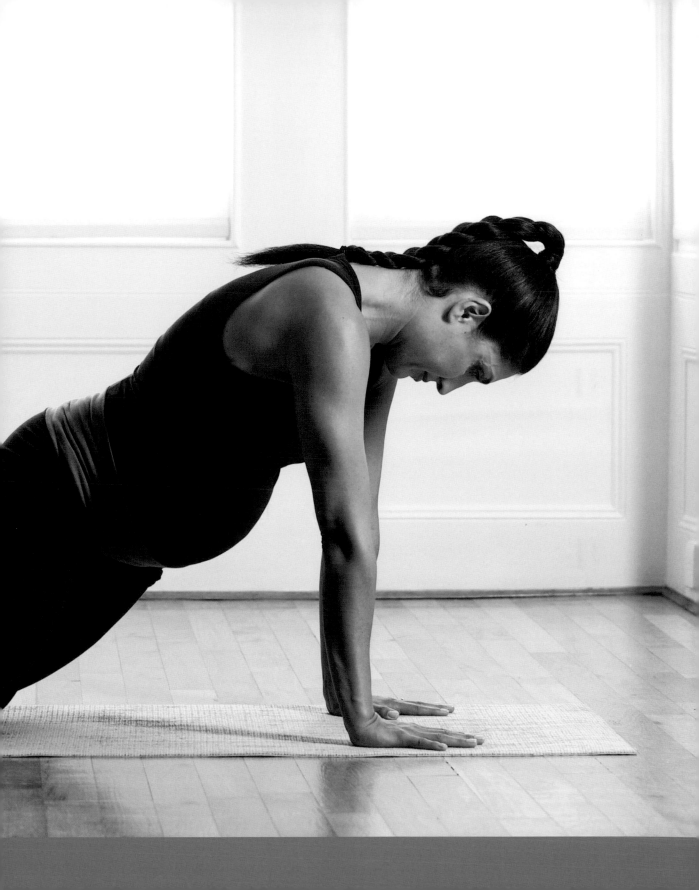

Affirmations

I am perfectly designed to give birth to my baby
— my body knows what to do.

My baby's birth will be easier if I stay
relaxed and breathe deeply.

I stay open-minded and go with the flow.

I see labour as an exciting challenge.

With each contraction I move a step closer
to meeting my baby.

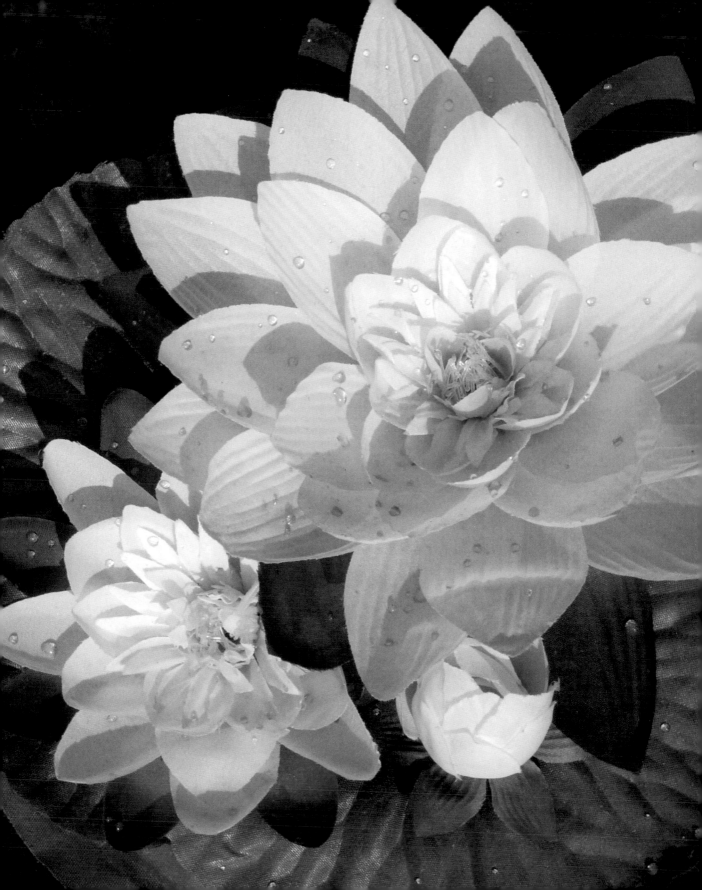

Preparing for Birth

You may know what kind of birth you would like to have, but keep an open mind as things usually don't go to plan. Complications can arise during labour and you may require an emergency caesarean. Whatever happens, remember that your yoga practice and breathing techniques will stand you in good stead. It is worth knowing exactly what a caesarean entails, even if you are planning to have a natural birth. In the event that you need a caesarean, it will be a less stressful experience for you if you understand the procedure. Read about it and, if possible, talk to someone who has been through the process. If you are having an elective caesarean, your yoga practice will have prepared your body well for recovery. You can still use breathing and visualization techniques, such as the Golden Thread Breath (see page 119).

On average babies arrive five days after their due date. Some doctors will insist on an induction once you are 7–10 days overdue. However, you can often ask to wait a few more days providing everything is fine with your baby and you are being monitored. You may be extremely uncomfortable toward the end of pregnancy as once the baby's head is engaged there is more pressure in your pelvis. Try to be patient and positive: consider these extra days a bonus, giving you more time to rest and nurture your baby in the womb. You may not feel like going too far from home, so doing gentle yoga exercises will help to keep you mobile and relieve nerves.

If you are overdue and your cervix is ready, your doctor may "sweep" the membranes to bring on labour. This and other procedures, such as having an internal examination, an epidural, or a catheter inserted, can be uncomfortable. It's helpful to practise your breathing techniques during these moments.

Yoga and meditation focus your attention on what is happening physically and light your inner life and your intuition. The ability to turn inward, allowing the thinking brain to switch off, is invaluable in coping with pain during labour. Most experts agree that if you are able to access your primitive self, move with your inner rhythms and lose your inhibitions, labour and birth can become much more manageable.

First-stage labour

The first stage of labour lasts from when the cervix starts to dilate through contractions to when you're ready to push and the cervix is around 10cm (4in) dilated. During this time it's good to remember your breathing. It will be your anchor throughout labour and birth. If you can keep your awareness focused on controlling your breath naturally and organically, your mind will remain calm.

Evidence suggests that being upright in the first stage results in less pain and less likelihood of needing an epidural, and ensures quicker progress to the second stage, so try to keep upright and move around during early labour. Walking, leaning against a wall or sitting with your arms resting on the back of a chair or on a birthing ball all help to speed up dilation, encourage contractions and allow your baby to descend farther into the pelvis. In the first stage, exercises on all fours, such as Cat (see pages 48–9), Hip Circles (see page 117) and Figure of Eight (see pages 122–3), are beneficial as they help position

Birth Story ...

"When my first baby was breech and I was advised to have a caesarean, I was incredibly disappointed as I had prepared so well for a natural birth. It took me a few weeks to get my head around the fact that as a pregnancy yoga teacher I wasn't going to be able to experience labour. However, once I had accepted this fact I decided to focus on all the positives of having a caesarean, such as knowing exactly what was going to happen and when. It was still an intimate and special occasion and my recovery was fast as I had prepared so well for the birth and I was fit and healthy." Tara Lee

your baby ready for the birth. Positions where your thighs are wide apart and the pelvic ligaments are stretched will give your baby more room to squeeze through the birth canal. For example, a squatting position – placing something underneath your heels is sometimes helpful – can open the pelvis by 30 percent more than when lying on your back. If you need to lie down, lie on your side. Better still, come into Child's Pose (see pages 80–81) or kneel on your bed while leaning forward.

Second-stage labour

This stage lasts from full dilation until you actually give birth, and you will have an overwhelming urge to bear down and push your baby out. As with the first stage of labour, if you are able to squat or be on all fours, gravity will assist you in pushing.

Using sounds is useful throughout labour but especially in the second stage. Sound lengthens the exhalation, giving the muscles more time to soften and release. It also helps the body to relax and open (see pages 24–5). The muscles in the jaw are connected to muscles in the cervix, so relaxing the jaw using these sounds can help to release the muscles around the cervix. Endorphins are released when you make sounds. They will help you to manage your pain. When you are in the second stage of labour, forcefully making the sound "G" (as in "Good" or "Great"), like a roar, imagining power behind the sound, may be very helpful for pushing your baby out into the world. You can also use "oooo" and "aaa" sounds resonating in the abdomen (see page 25). Imagine these sounds moving down through your body and out through the birth canal in a J-curve, moving your baby with them. Rest when you can between contractions to gather strength and focus, and try to keep your connection to the breath at all times.

Third-stage labour

The third stage of delivery is when the placenta is expelled. This may be managed naturally through contractions of the uterus or you may be offered an injection to speed up the process. Again, use your breathing techniques – slow deep breaths, focusing on the sound of the breath (see pages 24–5) – to help you through this process and also to manage the discomfort of any stitches and so on.

Hip Circles with Hands against the Wall

This exercise can help the baby's head drop farther down into the pelvis and is good to do in early labour.

1 Find a comfortable position leaning with your hands against the wall, making a pillow for your head. Keep your feet a little wider than hip-width apart and bend your knees.

2 Close your eyes and start to circle your hips. Let the movements be fluid and find your own rhythm. Make them big or small depending on how you feel.

3 Breathe deeply without forcing the breath and continue for as long as you like.

4 You can vary the movement by zig-zagging your hips from side to side.

5 Try to zig-zag down toward the ground and then back up again a few times, staying grounded through your feet, with knees bent.

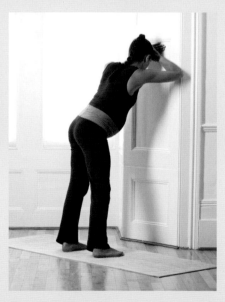

2

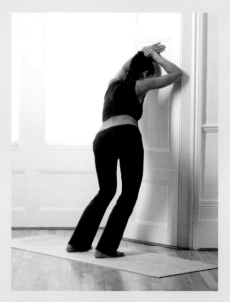

4

Ujjayi Breath

Ujjayi breathing is a technique used in regular yoga and is very useful to practise throughout pregnancy. Once you are familiar with it, you can use it in labour to help lower blood pressure and keep yourself calm.

1 Breathe in through your nose and breathe out of your mouth, placing your hand in front of your mouth. Keep your face relaxed and your eyes soft.

2 Close your mouth and try making the same sound with your breath. Focus on the sound of the breath to bring your attention within you – it should sound like the sea. Keep the breath fluid and regular. As you practise, your inhalation and exhalation should become longer and of similar quality.

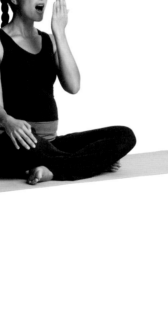

1

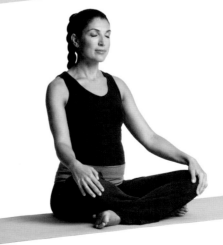

2

Golden Thread Breath

This is a wonderful way to combine breathing and visualization. It can be used whenever you need to feel calmer. It is an invaluable tool for labour when anxiety levels may rise and pain can begin to feel overwhelming. Holding this visual focus in your mind can carry you through, up and over the peak of each contraction.

1 Close your eyes and bring the thumb and index to touch in *jana mudra*. Inhale through your nose and, as you exhale, imagine there is a petal between your lips so they are slightly parted. Breathe out an imaginary golden thread into the distance.

2 Inhale through your nose and exhale through your mouth without forcing the breath. Imagine gently blowing this golden thread farther and farther into the distance, noticing how your exhalation gradually lengthens. PAUSE 🪷 Notice how much calmer you feel as you repeat this visualization with each breath.

- It may help you to imagine that this golden thread is like a golden rope helping you to climb to the top of a mountain – as your contraction reaches its peak this rope helps you to climb over the summit. You may also like to visualize sailing on the ocean holding onto this rope as it helps you to ride over the choppy waves.

3 Use these images in a relaxed way and see what works for you. Don't fight the waves – hold onto the golden rope so that you can ride them. Remember that there will be times of calm between the choppy waves when you can recoup your focus and energy so that you are ready for the next one.

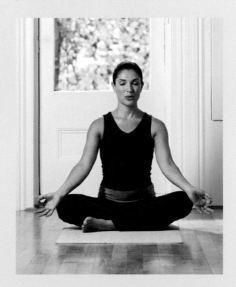

Rocking Back and Forth

Rocking back and forth can be done on all fours or on a birthing ball. This pose strengthens the arms, and helps to lubricate the hips and keep you mobile. It is good during labour as it gives your baby more space and encourages the head to move down into your pelvis ready for birth. Open your knees wider (unless you have groin pain) for stability and to give your baby even more room.

1 Rest your knees on the floor wide enough apart to feel a comfortable space for your baby. Lean forward and rest your arms on the ball.

2 As you inhale bring your weight forward onto your arms resting on the ball.

3 As you exhale move your weight back toward your heels, moving the ball as you do so. If you feel comfortable, increase the movement, moving your hips farther back toward your heels. Keep your head in line with your spine. Feel the movement through your entire body and feel supported by the ball.

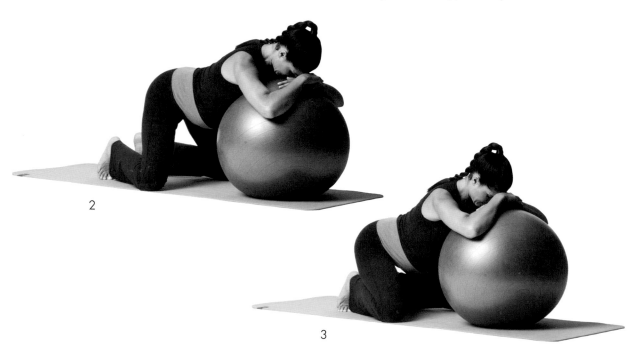

2

3

Hip Circles on the Ball

The following exercise also keeps a sense of fluidity through the hips and lessens the intensity of your contractions as you move. Remember always to breathe with long, deep, relaxed inhalations and exhalations. This will help your baby to move down into the pelvis ready for birth. Performing these circles throughout your pregnancy will assist in releasing tightness from the hips.

1 Make sure that your feet are pressing firmly into the floor, hip-width or wider apart for support, and that you are sitting evenly on the ball.

2 Keep the breath flowing freely as you move your hips to the left.

3 Make a circle, coming back to the centre and moving your hips to the right. Keep moving fluidly, finding your own rhythm and making the circles as big or as small as feels comfortable. Use the movement to release any tightness from your hips.

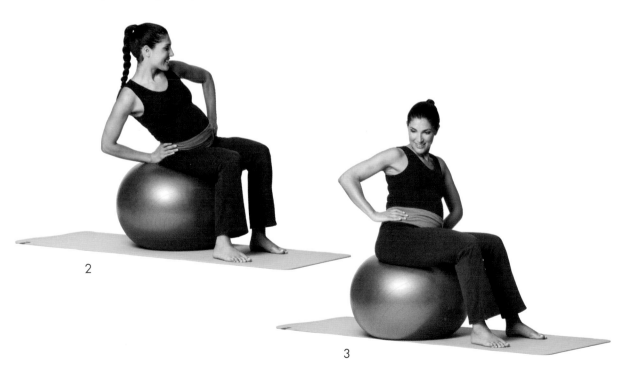

2

3

Figure of Eight

This builds on other hip-circling exercises you have learned. It is one of the best exercises to use during contractions and helps the baby move into an optimal position for birth. Your baby has to rotate to travel out of the birth canal. Remember your breath – keep it flowing. Don't hold it or your muscles will tighten. Allow your breath to flow with each contraction. Breathe through these surges, riding the wave over its peak until it subsides.

1 From an all-fours position, start by moving your pelvis in small circles, gradually letting them get bigger, as if you are having an internal dance with your baby. Close your eyes and tune in to how your body is feeling as you move, keeping your knuckles pressing down, your fingers spread, and the tops of your feet pressing into the floor. If you need to, widen your knees to feel more stable.

2 Slow down the circling and gradually come back to the centre. Check your position and make sure the weight is still even in both hands and knees.

3 Now start to make small circles in the other direction and gradually increase them if this feels comfortable.

4 Vary the circles adding a figure of eight. Again, you can make this as small or as large as feels comfortable. Imagine freeing up any areas of tightness as you breathe into the movement, keeping it as fluid as possible, moving at your own pace.

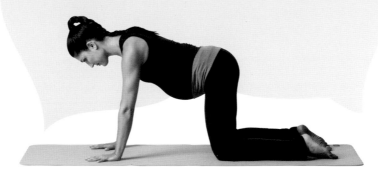

1

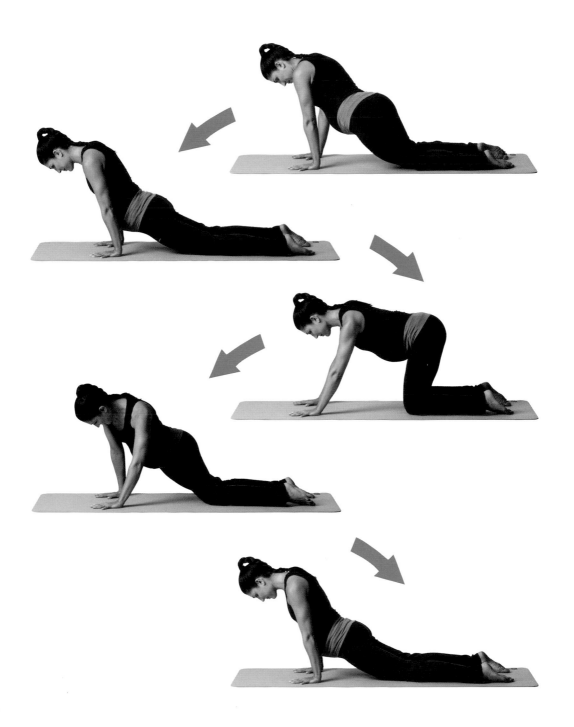

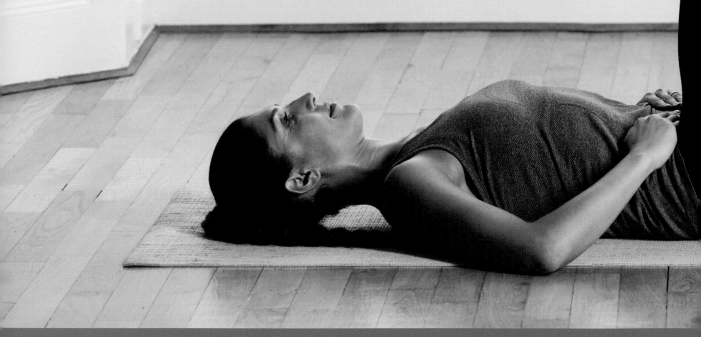
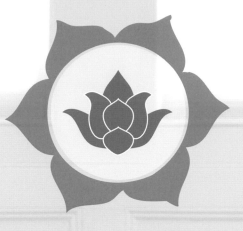

CHAPTER 7
Getting Back in Shape

Now that your baby has arrived, everything has changed and getting to yoga classes may not be easy. However, this is a time when you are likely to need yoga more than ever. Although most of your days are spent looking after your newborn, you also need to nurture yourself. The following exercises will help you to do just that by releasing tension, improving your body image and giving you some much-needed energy.

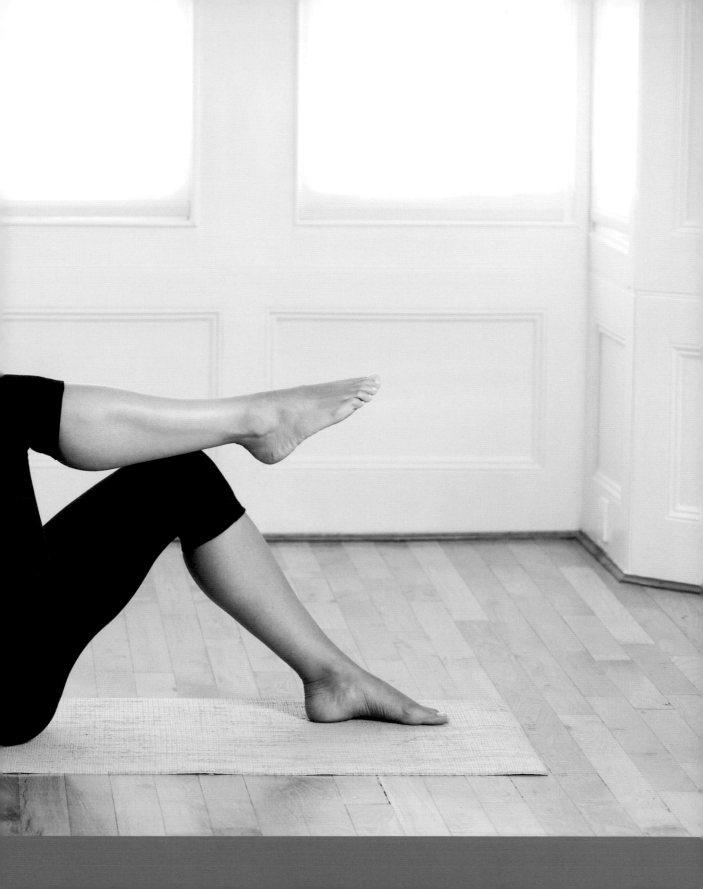

Affirmations

The first few months may be difficult but
I will get my life back again!

I remain centred and relaxed, regardless
of what is happening around me.

I am letting go of the need to control.

I will rest whenever I can and not put too
many expectations on myself.

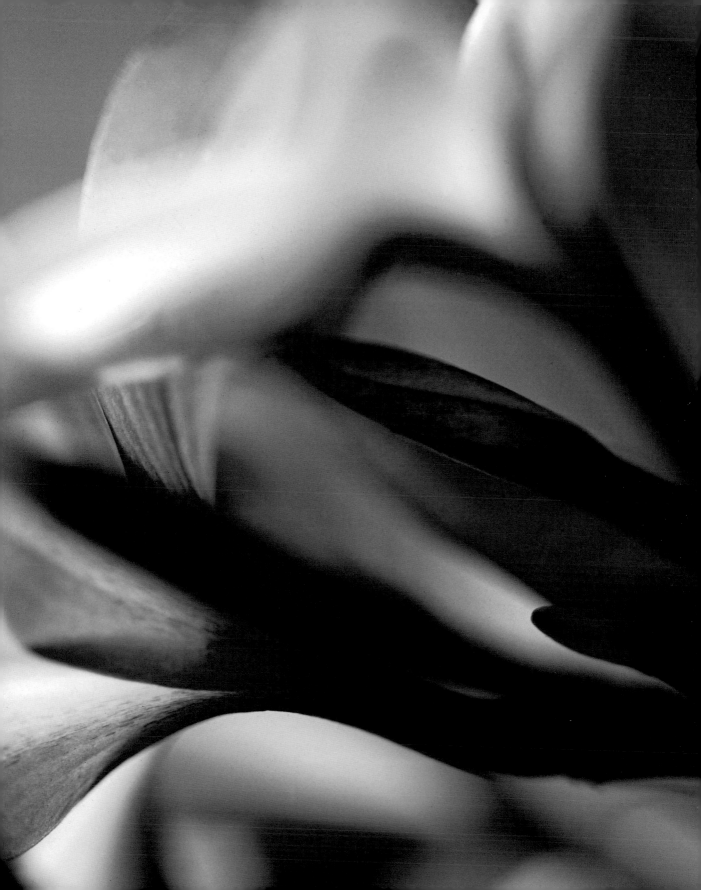

After the Birth of Your Baby

Your body has been through nine months of immense changes. Be respectful of this. It may take time to rebuild your strength and confidence. If you can, remain as still and as centred as possible in the first few weeks as this will make you feel restored and better able to adjust to your baby's demands and the major changes in your life. I recommend starting exercise six weeks after the birth (after your postnatal check-up), but you can focus on relaxation and meditation immediately whenever you have spare time. If you have had a caesarean, wait for 12 weeks or until you have had the all-clear from your doctor. Remember to take all exercise gently as you will still have high levels of the hormone relaxin in your body and it is easier to overstretch.

The recti muscles are two large muscle sheets that cover the internal organs in the abdomen, meeting in the middle of the abdomen. Toward the end of pregnancy, these abdominal muscles can separate (a condition known as diastasis recti), to make more space for your baby, leaving a gap. Many women feel discomfort in the last weeks of pregnancy as this separation occurs. This discomfort usually subsides after a few days. However, in some cases the gap can continue to widen over time. To check whether you have any separation, lie on your back and lift your shoulders off the floor. Holding your index and third finger vertically, press horizontally, starting at the top of the recti muscles (at your sternum/breastbone), and work your way down toward your belly button and pubic bone. If the gap is sufficiently wide that both your fingers descend into it, you should get checked by your doctor or physiotherapist to see if you have diastasis recti. If you see a doming at your midline when you get out of bed or the bath, this may also be a sign. Gentle postnatal abdominal exercises can strengthen the abdominal muscles, helping them eventually to "knit" back together again. If left untreated, separated muscles can lead to pelvic instability, lower back pain and altered posture, so it is important to do the exercises that are recommended by your doctor or physiotherapist. Strong abdominal exercises such as crunches should be avoided if you have diastasis recti as they can worsen the condition.

Yoga is a wonderful way of releasing the tension in the upper back and shoulders that can build from carrying and feeding your baby. Developing core strength is important for preventing back pain. Doing cardiovascular exercise also releases endorphins, which will improve your emotional state. And yoga can help you to bond with your baby, making you feel more positive about yourself, improving your body image and helping you to deal with the big change in your life.

Approach this whole new chapter in your life with compassion for yourself. Enjoy seeing your baby growing and developing each day. Go with the flow. It is not unusual to feel very emotional. This is often a sign that your hormones are fluctuating, but can also be a sign that you are exhausted. Make sure you are eating well and, when possible, try to nap at the same time as your baby. Join mother-and-baby groups, meet friends and get plenty of fresh air. Above all, don't be too tough on yourself, or try to do it all, or compare yourself and your baby with others. It is very important to allow your partner or husband the chance to get to know your baby, develop confidence and discover their own way of looking after the child, which may be different from yours. It's good for you to have some time off from caring for your baby and this also really helps to cement the relationship between father and baby.

Making time for yoga practice will remind you that it's not necessary to hold your baby all the time – it will be fine in its own company, with you present or nearby. As long as your baby is not unsettled or distressed, it is healthy for both of you to have some space of your own. Your baby will learn to feel secure if you encourage some independence. This can be very liberating. Listen to your intuition and be guided by this, and be aware that habits you create with your baby are quick to develop and hard to break!

It is important to establish a sense of balance and some sort of routine in your life with a new baby. There's no escaping the fact that initially your life will revolve around your newborn and that you will not have much time for yourself. You can start by doing a little bit of yoga whenever you manage to find a moment. It may only be five minutes but it will help to make you feel more energized and release tightness from your body. Over time you can build up your practice and you should find your strength and energy start to return. Any of the exercises in this book are appropriate when you feel ready, but the following postures are designed specifically for postnatal recovery. Remember, there's no rush to get back in shape – after all, your body has been through nine months of upheaval. Be patient. It may take a while for your body and energy to return to normal, but you will get there in the end!

Birth Story ...

"Little Luke is now four months old and he's doing really well. My body is getting back on track, which I think is down to all the yoga I did during my pregnancy, and the postnatal exercises seem to be really helping me. I'm amazed at my recovery and how my strength is coming back! It took a while until I had enough energy to feel like doing yoga again, but as soon as I began, I felt so much better. I hadn't realized how tight and achy my body had become! I started slowly and now aim to do just 5–10 minutes nearly every day, but I sometimes manage 30 minutes on a good day! It feels so good for my body to stretch and breathe deeply, and afterwards I feel refreshed, calm and better able to deal with my baby – even when I am exhausted! Life is very different now, I'm having to juggle a lot more and there are days when I don't manage to get out of my pyjamas, but I'm trying not to worry about getting much done during the day. I think the yoga and becoming a mother have taught me not to put too much pressure on myself and to live more in the moment. I'm really enjoying the time I have with Luke as I know each stage passes so quickly and I will be going back to part-time work soon." Jodie

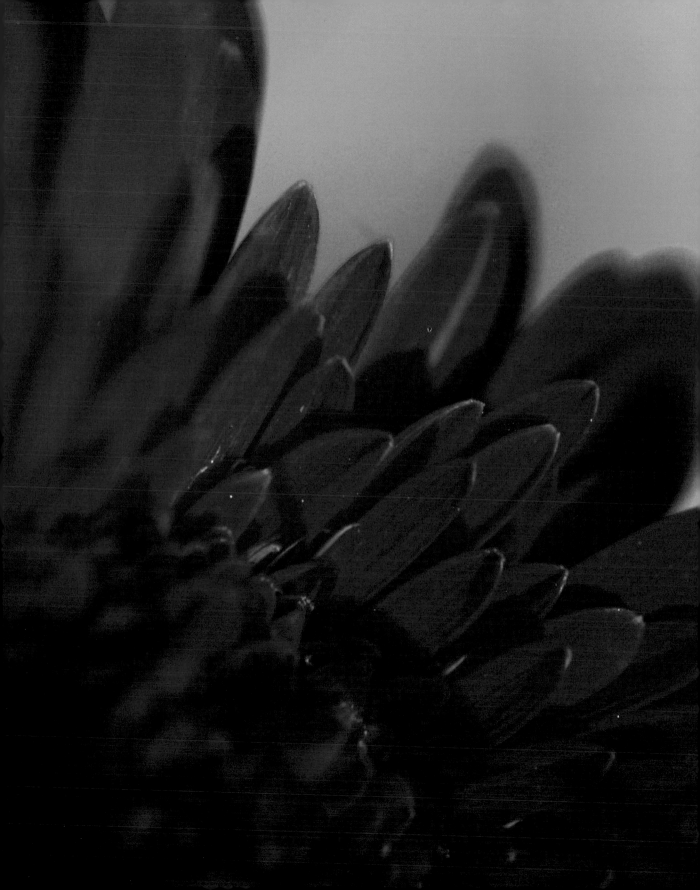

Drawing Circles in Side Stretch

Side stretches are a wonderful way to open up the lungs. On a physical level, this helps to decompress the whole chest cavity. On an emotional and spiritual level, the lungs are seen in yoga theory as the seat of the soul. It is always good to connect to this area when there are external demands in your life.

1 Place your left hand on the floor, palm flat and fingers away from you. Extend your right arm in line with your ear without hunching your shoulder. Feel the stretch down the side of your body as you continue to reach over farther.

2 Bend your left elbow and inhale, breathing into your side.

3 Still on the out-breath, sweep your right arm across the floor in front of you.

4 Inhale as your arm comes around and back up – imagine that you have a paintbrush on the end of your fingers and you are seeing how big you can paint the circles. Try to follow your arm with your gaze.

5 Make 5 big sweeping circles and then repeat with the other arm to the other side.

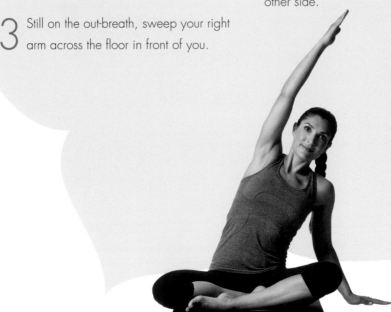

1

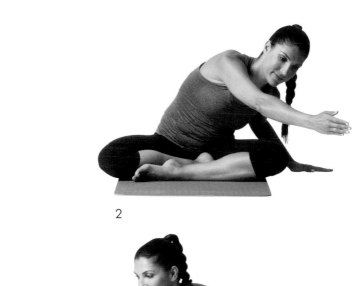

2

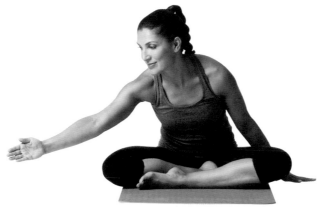

3

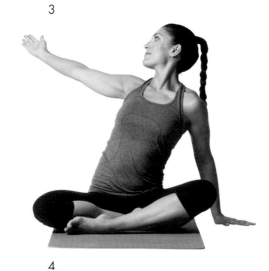

4

Lower Abs Strengthening

This strengthens the abs and can help them to knit back together. If you have abdominal separation (see page 128), see your doctor and start from Step 3.

1 Sit with feet parallel and hip-width apart. Straighten your arms and adjust your feet so your fingers can touch your heels. Rest your hands in front of your knees, keeping your buttocks on the floor, your shoulders and neck relaxed, and your hips and chest gently lifted.

2 Keeping your feet pressing into the floor, exhale, release your hands and roll down slowly through the lower, middle, then upper back.

3 Now, lying on your back with your hands down by your sides, ensure that your hips are even, your pubic bone is in line with your navel, your shoulders are relaxed, and your chin is tucked in.

4 Inhale, taking the breath from the base of your spine to the top. Exhaling, use your pelvic floor to lift your right leg, keeping the knee bent at a right-angle and making sure not to arch your back.

5 Inhale through your nose and as you exhale out of your mouth slowly lower your leg, feeling your core control the move. At the same time soften your ribs and neck and relax your shoulders. Repeat for your left leg. Continuing to take turns, lift each leg 3–5 times.

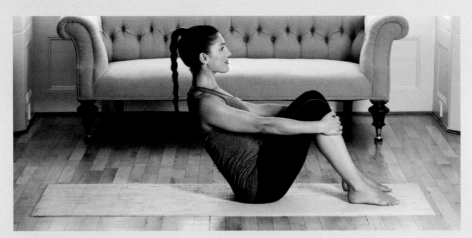

1

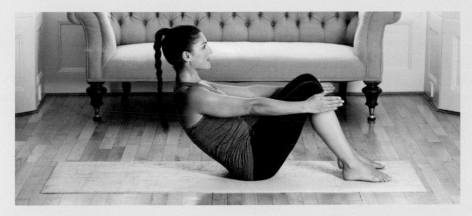

2

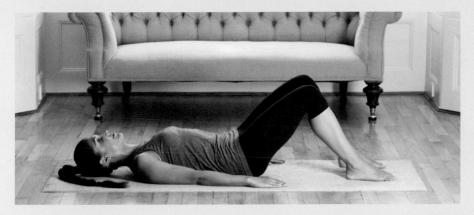

3

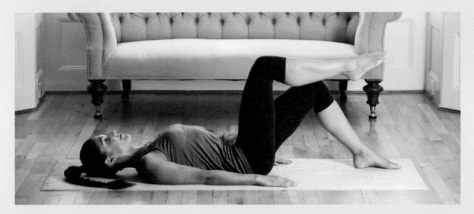

4

Inner Thigh Strengthening

This exercise is great on many levels. It strengthens your pelvic floor and inner thighs, helps to realign your spine, and engages your core. This can also be a useful exercise for backache.

1 Place a pillow between your knees and squeeze gently. Inhale, taking the breath gently into your upper back.

2 As you exhale start to roll your hips in toward you, peeling your hips away from the mat. Lift through your lower, middle and upper back, softening your ribs as you lift. Feel your centre and pelvic floor switch on, and push gently through your feet, lifting as high as you can. Keep squeezing your cushion.

3 Inhale and as you exhale, lift your arms back over your head without arching your neck. Feel your body lengthen.

4 Inhale and as you exhale lift the arms toward the ceiling.

5 Inhale and slowly unravel your spine – the upper, the middle and then the lower back – releasing back down into the floor and placing your arms by your sides, with palms down (as Step 1).

6 Repeat 3–5 times, inhaling, and then as you exhale lifting your arms and hips, letting the movement flow. Inhale and exhale, and roll back down through each vertebra, releasing tension as you go. Finally, relax for a few minutes.

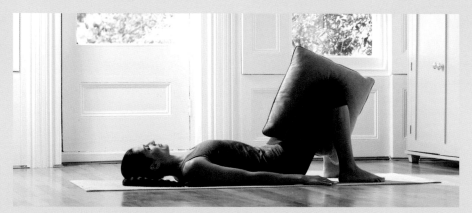

1

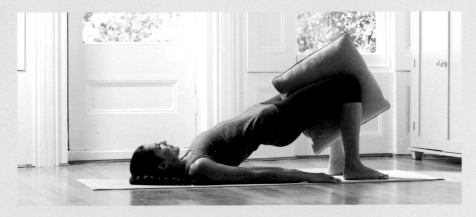

2

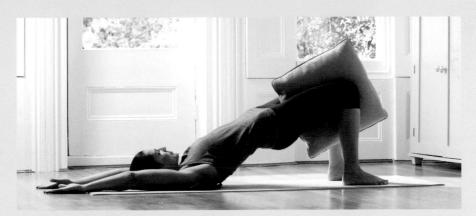

3

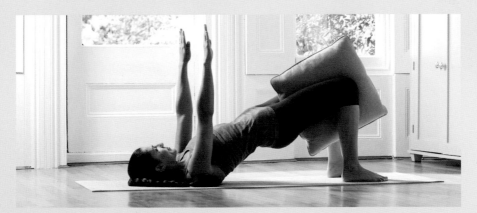

4

Table

This exercise will strengthen your arms and legs and at the same time open up the front of your shoulders and chest – much needed after all the feeding and carrying you are doing.

1 Sit on the floor with knees bent and place your hands behind you, fingers facing forward, spread out. Squeeze your shoulder blades toward each other and relax your shoulders down.

2 Pressing through your hands and feet, use the strength in your legs to lift your hips as high as you can, squeezing and engaging your pelvic floor muscles. If your tummy is popping out, tilt your pelvis slightly in and draw your pelvic floor muscles up and in while engaging your abdominal muscles.

If you are finding this exercise difficult, try to do it sitting on the floor with your legs crossed, or kneeling, or place a book or block underneath your hands to raise the level of your hands from the mat. Keep the fronts of your shins pressing straight ahead.

3 Release your head back gently (or if you prefer, keep looking forward) and stay for up to 5 breaths, breathing deeply. Bring your head back up to look forward and exhale slowly, lowering back down to the floor.

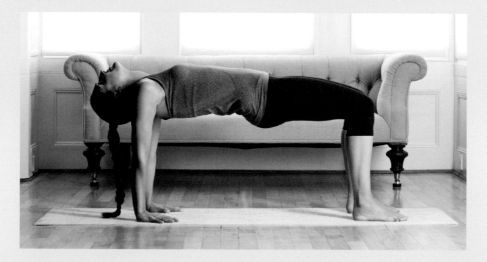

Locust

This exercise can energize you if you are feeling tired. It strengthens the lower back while opening the front body and can help to improve your posture and relieve lower back pain. Although you no longer have to contend with the weight of your baby in your womb, this is still a time in your life when your back is likely to be under more strain than normal!

For comfort you may prefer to place a folded blanket beneath your ribs while practising this pose.

1 Lying on your abdomen, interlace your fingers behind your back, drawing your arms back to lift your head and shoulders away from the mat. Firm your buttocks and keep squeezing your shoulder blades toward each other. Lengthen your legs away from you on the floor. Gaze forward, keeping the back of your neck long. PAUSE 🪷

- If you find this too much, place your hands under your shoulders and press into your hands to lift your chest (shoulders drawing down and back).

2 Hold for up to 5 slow breaths and focus on drawing your abdominal muscles in and keeping them steady for support.

3 Exhale and slowly release back down again. Make a pillow with your hands and rest your head down. Notice if your shoulders feel freer, and breathe into your upper back.

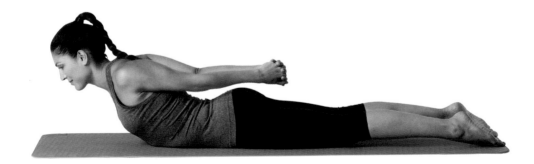

Lower Back Strengthening

This is a great exercise for strengthening the pelvic floor, helping to build strength in your lower back and drawing all your abdominal muscles back into their pre-pregnancy positions.

1 Lie on your stomach. Place your arms out in front, shoulder-width apart, shoulders down, lengthening through your legs. Keep your chin tucked in and your hips square.

2 Inhale, and as you exhale raise your right arm and left leg off the floor. At the same time lift your head, keeping your neck long and your gaze down toward the floor. Feel your centre gently lift away from the mat, and soften your ribs, trying not to tilt your

hips. Lengthening and broadening through the back of the knee, working from your centre, keep your arm long, reaching through your fingers.

3 Inhale once more, taking your breath all the way into your upper back, and as you exhale really be aware of your pelvic floor lifting.

4 Return to the starting position, then repeat with the other arm and leg. Repeat 3 times on each side.

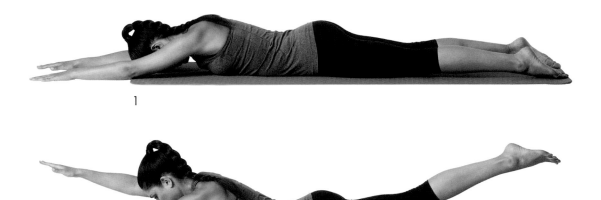

1

2

Leg Slides

This exercise helps you to engage and gently restore strength in the abdominal muscles. It is good for encouraging the muscles to come back together if you have had any abdominal separation (see page 128).

1 Lie on your back with your knees bent and feet hip-width apart and parallel. Inhale, and as you exhale draw your navel in about 30 percent toward your spine, engaging your abdominal muscles. Feel your lower back pressing toward the floor.

2 Try to keep your muscles engaged, maintaining this core activation, as you slowly slide your right leg away from you, keeping your back still.

3 Inhale and bring your right leg back to the start position. (You can place your hands on your abdomen to make sure you are drawing your muscles toward your spine and possibly feel your muscles switching on.) Repeat with the other leg. Try this 5 times on each leg.

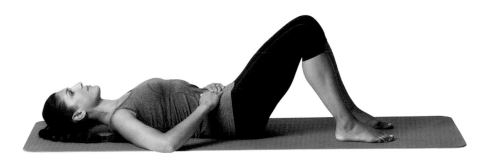

1

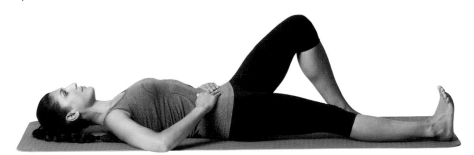

2

Index

Using the DVD

The DVD that accompanies this book is a 30-minute restorative yoga practice, which will help to bring you back to a sense of wholeness, allowing you to feel centred and empowered. Focusing on deep, calming breathing exercises and gentle, restorative poses, it can be used any time from 12–14 weeks of pregnancy to help release tension in the body and the mind. The exercises shown on the DVD are described in the book on the following pages:

0:28 *Pranayama* pp.18–20

5:20 Foot Circling p.109

6:39 Leaning Back into Hands pp.104–5

7:15 Child's Pose pp.80–81

8:20 Side Stretches p.36

9:47 Rounding and Straightening p.92

11:45 Cow-faced Pose p.103

13:03 Cat and Swooping Cat pp.48–9

15:01 Strengthening the Pelvic Floor pp.50–51

17:22 Figure of Eight pp.122–3

19:28 Pigeon p.106

21:31 *Tadasana* p.55

22:39 Arm Swinging p.41

23:33 Wide-legged Forward Bend p.56

25:44 Tree p.57

27:27 Leaning on a Chair/Wall p.78

28:47 *Savasana* pp.84–5

Acknowledgments

Tara Lee My thanks must go to my husband Inigo for all his support and patience when I was writing this book and to our two children for continuing to inspire and teach me. Thank you to my students, from whom I never stop learning.

Mary Attwood I would like to thank my son, without whom I could not have made this journey and who provided me with so many lasting insights during my own pregnancy – and who continues to inspire me.

Tara's cushioned "Bump" pregnancy yoga mat and her "Bump, Birth & Beyond" DVD boxset are available now at taraleeyoga.com